ACT Prep Study Guide 2015-2016

Table of Contents

INTRODUCTION 5
GETTING READY FOR TEST DAY 6
GENERAL STRATEGIES 7
    STRATEGY 1: UNDERSTANDING THE INTIMIDATION 7
    STRATEGY 2: FINDING YOUR OPTIMAL PACE 7
    STRATEGY 3: DON'T BE A PERFECTIONIST 7
    STRATEGY 4: FACTUALLY CORRECT, BUT ACTUALLY WRONG 8
    STRATEGY 5: EXTRANEOUS INFORMATION 8
    STRATEGY 6: AVOIDING DEFINITES 8
    STRATEGY 7: USING COMMON SENSE 8
    STRATEGY 8: INSTINCTS ARE RIGHT 9
    STRATEGY 9: NO FEAR 9
    STRATEGY 10: DON'T GET THROWN OFF BY NEW INFORMATION 9
    STRATEGY 11: NARROWING THE SEARCH 9
    STRATEGY 12: YOU'RE NOT EXPECTED TO BE EINSTEIN 9

THE ENGLISH TEST 10
    SIMPLICITY IS BLISS 10
    PARALLELISM 10
    GRAMMAR TYPE 10
    PUNCTUATION 11
    TENSE 11
    ADDED PHRASES 11
    WORD CONFUSION 12
        Contractions 12
        Its/It's 12
        They're/Their/There 12
        Who's/Whose 13
        Their/His 13
        That/Who 13
        Who/Whom or Whoever/Whomever 13
        Correct Pronoun Usage in Combinations 14
    COMMAS 14
        Flow 14
        Nonessential Clauses and Phrases 14
        Subjects and Verbs 15

> *Independent Clauses* *15*
> *Parenthetical Expressions* *16*
> *Sentence Beginnings* *16*

HYPHENS 16
SEMICOLONS 16

> *Period Replacement* *16*
> *Related/Unrelated* *17*
> *Comparative Methods of Joining Clauses* *17*
> *Transitions* *17*
> *Items in a Series* *17*

PARENTHESES 17

> *Years* *17*
> *Nonessential Information* *18*
> *Items in a Series* *18*
> *Independent Clauses* *18*

APOSTROPHES 18

THE MATH TEST 19

PRE-ALGEBRA AND ALGEBRA 19
TRIGONOMETRY 36

THE READING TEST 42

COMPREHENSION SKILLS 42
TESTING TIPS 52

> *Skimming* *52*
> *Paragraph Focus* *53*
> *Eliminate Choices* *54*
> *Contextual Clues* *54*
> *Fact/Opinion* *55*
> *Time Management* *55*
> *Warnings* *55*

THE SCIENCE REASONING TEST 57

FOUR TYPES OF PASSAGES 57
FOUR TYPES OF QUESTIONS 58
ANSWER CHOICE ELIMINATION TECHNIQUES 58

> *Informal Language* *58*
> *Extreme Statements* *58*
> *Similar Answer Choices* *59*

TIME MANAGEMENT	59
HIGHLY TECHNICAL QUESTIONS MAY NOT BE	60
EXPERIMENT PASSAGES	60
RANDOM TIPS	61

THE WRITING TEST 62

Brainstorm	*62*
Strength through Diversity	*62*
Pick a Main Idea	*62*
Weed the Garden	*62*
Create a Logical Flow	*63*
Start Your Engines	*63*
First Paragraph	*63*
Body Paragraph	*63*
Conclusion Paragraph	*63*
Don't Panic	*63*
Check Your Work	*64*
FINAL NOTE	64

APPENDIX A: TIME STATISTICS FOR THE ACT 65
APPENDIX B: SAT/ACT EQUIVALENCY TABLE 66
APPENDIX C: AREA, VOLUME, SURFACE AREA FORMULAS 67
APPENDIX D: PRACTICE TEST 68

ENGLISH	68
MATHEMATICS	79
READING	89
SCIENCE	97

ANSWER KEY AND EXPLANATIONS 106

ENGLISH	106
MATHEMATICS	110
READING	114
SCIENCE	117

Introduction

The purpose of the exam is to establish a standard method of measurement for the skills and abilities that have been acquired by the test taker. These skills are both a measure of what a test taker has already learned and an indicator of future success.

The exam requires you to think in a thorough, quick and strategic manner, and still be accurate, logical and wise. It is designed to judge your abilities in the ways that the testing organization feel is vital to your future success.

To some extent, you have already gradually obtained these abilities over the length of your academic career. However, what you probably have not yet become familiar with is the capability to use these abilities for the purpose of maximizing performance within the complex and profound environment of a standardized, skills-based examination.

There are different strategies, mindsets and perspectives that you will be required to apply throughout the exam. You'll need to be prepared to use your whole brain as far as thinking and assessment is concerned, and you'll need to do this in a timely manner. This is not something you can learn from taking a course or reading a book, but it is something you can develop through practice and concentration.

Fortunately, the exam does not change very dramatically from year to year. This makes it a little easier to prepare knowing that any information you use to prepare with should still be accurate when you go to take the test.

The following information in this guide will lay out the format and style of the exam as well as help prepare you for the frame of mind you'll be expected to take. If there is one skill that you take with you from your exam preparation, this should be it.

Careful preparation, as described in this expert guide, along with hard work, will dramatically enhance your probability of success. In fact, it is wise to apply this philosophy not only to your exam, but to other elements of your life as well, to raise you above the competition.

Your exam score is so important to your future success that it should not be taken lightly. Hence, a rational, prepared approach to your exam is critical.

Keep in mind, that although it may be possible to take the exam more than once, you should never take it as an "experiment" just to see how well you do. It is of extreme importance that you always be prepared to do your best when taking the exam. For one thing, it is extremely challenging to surmount a poor performance. If you are looking to take a "practice" run, look into a review course, practice tests, and, of course, this guide.

This guide provides you with the professional instruction you require for understanding the test. Covered are all aspects of the test and preparation procedures that you will require throughout the process. Upon completion of this guide, you'll have the confidence and knowledge you need for maximizing your exam performance.

Getting Ready For Test Day

You're all set to take your exam! Now here are a few things to remember for test day:

Get there early. Know exactly where the test will be held and how you will get yourself there. Pay attention to traffic reports so that you can compensate for any unexpected issues on the road. Leaving early will mean that you'll be more relaxed; red traffic lights won't raise your stress level, and you won't be pulled over by the first officer who has to fill his speeding ticket quota. Finally, and perhaps most importantly, you'll have time to use the rest room.

If you've got butterflies in your stomach, feed them! You've already done all the practice tests you can do, and you've had a good night's sleep. Now it's time to get a good, healthy breakfast - though it is wise not to overeat. Your body and mind will need the energy; plus it's distracting to listen to your stomach growl.

Give yourself a massage! Rub your head, neck and shoulders. Place your hand over your heart while taking a very slow, deep breath.

Stay on track. Remember, you don't want to rush, you only want to perform in a timely manner. Although there are time restrictions, if you misread directions, accidentally fill in the wrong answer-choice, or think illogically due to rushing, it won't be worth all the time you save. Remember, haste makes waste! Also, keep in mind that incorrect answers don't count against you, so you can always guess at any answers that you are unsure of. Remember, an educated guess is better than no guess at all! Moving through a test methodically and efficiently will likely mean that you'll have more time at the end than if you were to rush and stumble, or dawdle over questions that you're struggling with.

Most importantly (at least to your sanity), remember that once it's over, it's over. Clear your mind of it, because you did your best. Go treat yourself to a hot chocolate or an ice cream cone, catch a movie with some friends and relax!

General Strategies

Strategy 1: Understanding the Intimidation

The test writers will generally choose some material on the exam that will be completely foreign to most test takers. You can't expect all of the topics to be ones with which you have a fair amount of familiarity. If you do happen to come across a high number of topics that you are extremely familiar with, consider yourself lucky, but don't plan on that happening.

In going through each question, try and understand all of the material at your disposal, while weeding out the distracter information. Note that you won't have a nice title overhead explaining the general topic being covered but will immediately be thrown into the middle of a strange format that you don't recognize.

Getting hit by strange sounding topics that you don't recognize, of which you may only have a small exposure, is just normal on the exam. Just remember that the questions themselves will contain all the information necessary to choose a correct answer.

Strategy 2: Finding your Optimal Pace

Everyone reads and tests at a different rate. It will take practice to determine what is the optimal rate at which you can read fast and yet absorb and comprehend the information.

With practice, you will find the pace that you should maintain on the test while answering the questions. It should be a comfortable rate. This is not a speed-reading test. If you have a good pace, and don't spend too much time on any question, you should have a sufficient amount of time to read the questions at a comfortable rate. The two extremes you want to avoid are the dumbfounded mode, in which you are lip reading every word individually and mouthing each word as though in a stupor, and the overwhelmed mode, where you are panicked and are buzzing back and forth through the question in a frenzy and not comprehending anything.

You must find your own pace that is relaxed and focused, allowing you to have time for every question and give you optimal comprehension. Note that you are looking for optimal comprehension, not maximum comprehension. If you spent hours on each word and memorized the question, you would have maximum comprehension. That isn't the goal though, you want to optimize how much you comprehend with how much time you spend reading each question. Practice will allow you to determine that optimal rate.

Strategy 3: Don't be a Perfectionist

If you're a perfectionist, this may be one of the hardest strategies, and yet one of the most important. The test you are taking is timed, and you cannot afford to spend too much time on any one question.

If you are working on a question and you've got your answer split between two possible answer choices, and you're going back through the question and reading it over and over again in order to decide between the two answer choices, you can be in one of the most frustrating situations possible. You feel that if you just spent one more minute on the problem, that you would be able to figure the right answer out and decide between the two. Watch out! You can easily get so absorbed in that problem that you loose track of time, get off track and end up spending the rest of the test playing catch up because of all the wasted time, which may leave you rattled and cause you to miss even more questions that you would have otherwise.

Therefore, unless you will only be satisfied with a perfect score and your abilities are in the top .1% strata of test takers, you should not go into the test with the mindset that you've got to get every question right. It is far better to accept that you will have to guess on some questions and possibly get them wrong and still have time for every question, than to analyze every question until you're absolutely confident in your answer and then run out of time on the test.

Strategy 4: Factually Correct, but Actually Wrong

A favorite ploy of question writers is to write answer choices that are factually correct on their own, but fail to answer the question, and so are actually wrong.

When you are going through the answer choices and one jumps out for being factually correct, watch out. Before you mark it as your answer choice, first make sure that you go back to the question and confirm that the answer choice answers the question being asked.

Strategy 5: Extraneous Information

Some answer choices will seem to fit in and answer the question being asked. They might even be factually correct. Everything seems to check out, so what could possibly be wrong?

Does the answer choice actually match the question, or is it based on extraneous information contained in the question. Just because an answer choice seems right, don't assume that you overlooked information while reading the question. Your mind can easily play tricks on you and make you think that you read something or that you overlooked a phrase.

Unless you are behind on time, always go back to the question and make sure that the answer choice "checks out."

Strategy 6: Avoiding Definites

Answer choices that make definite statements with no "wiggle room" are often wrong. Try to choose answer choices that make less definite and more general statements that would likely be correct in a wider range of situations and aren't exclusive.

Answer choices that includes phrases like "sometimes" or "often" are more likely to be correct than answer choices with phrases like "always" or "never".

Strategy 7: Using Common Sense

The questions on the test are not intended to be trick questions. Therefore, most of the answer choices will have a sense of normalcy about them that may be fairly obvious and could be answered simply by using common sense.

While many of the topics will be ones that you are somewhat unfamiliar with, there will likely be numerous topics that you have some prior indirect knowledge about that will help you answer the questions.

Strategy 8: Instincts are Right

When in doubt, go with your first instinct. This is an old test-taking trick that still works today. Oftentimes if something feels right instinctively, it is right. Unfortunately, over analytical test takers will often convince themselves otherwise. Don't fall for that trap and try not to get too nitpicky about an answer choice. You shouldn't have to twist the facts and create hypothetical scenarios for an answer choice to be correct.

Strategy 9: No Fear

The depth and breadth of the exam can be a bit intimidating to a lot of people as it can deal with topics that have never been encountered before and are highly technical. Don't get bogged down by the information presented. Don't try to understand every facet of every question. You won't have to write an essay about the topics afterwards, so don't memorize all of the minute details. Don't get overwhelmed.

Strategy 10: Don't Get Thrown Off by New Information

Sometimes test writers will include completely new information in answer choices that are wrong. Test takers will get thrown off by the new information and if it seems like it might be related, they could choose that answer choice incorrectly. Make sure that you don't get distracted by answer choices containing new information that doesn't answer the question.

If an answer choice asks about something that wasn't even mentioned elsewhere, it's likely wrong. There has to be a connection between the answer choice and the question.

Strategy 11: Narrowing the Search

Whenever two answer choices are direct opposites, the correct answer choice is usually one of the two. It is hard for test writers to resist making one of the wrong answer choices with the same wording, but changing one word to make it the direct opposite in meaning. This can usually cue a test taker in that one of the two choices is correct. You can typically rule out the other answer choices.

Strategy 12: You're not Expected to be Einstein

The questions will contain most or all of the information that you need to know in order to answer them. You aren't expected to be Einstein or to know all related knowledge to the topic being discussed. Remember, these questions may be about obscure topics that you've never heard of. If you would need to know a lot of outside and background knowledge about a topic in order to choose a certain answer choice – it's usually wrong.

The English Test

The English portion of the ACT will have questions about underlined portions of text, with possible replacements as answer choices. Read the text four times, each time replacing the underlined portion with one of the choices. While reading the choices, read the sentence before, the sentence containing, and the sentence after the underlined portion. Sometimes an answer may make sense until you read the following sentence and see how the two sentences flow together. While reading the text, be sure to pause at each comma. If the comma is necessary the pause will be logical. If the comma is not needed, then the sentence will feel awkward. Transitional words should create smooth, logical transitions and maintain a constant flow of text.

Some questions will be concerning sentence insertions. In those cases, do not look for the ones that simply restate what was in the previous sentence. New sentences should contain new information and new insights into the subject of the text. If asked for the paragraph to which a sentence would most naturally be added, find a key noun or word in that new sentence. Then find the paragraph containing that exact word, or another word closely related to that key noun or word. That is the paragraph that should include the new sentence.

Some questions will ask what purpose a phrase fulfilled in a particular text. It depends upon the subject of the text. If the text is dramatic, then the phrase was probably used to show tension. If the text is comedic, then the phrase may have been there to relieve tension.

In related cases, you may be asked to provide a sentence that summarizes the text. Simple sentences, without wordy phrases, are usually best. If asked for a succinct answer, then the shorter the answer, the more likely it is correct.

Simplicity Is Bliss

Simplicity cannot be overstated. You should never choose a longer, more complicated, or wordier replacement if a simple one will do. When a point can be made with fewer words, choose that answer. However, never sacrifice the flow of text for simplicity. If an answer is simple, but does not make sense, then it is not correct.

Beware of added phrases that don't add anything of meaning, such as *to be* or *as to them*. Often these added phrases will occur just before a colon, which may come before a list of items. However, the colon does not need a lengthy introduction. The phrases after the comma in the examples below are wordy and unnecessary. They should be removed and the colon placed directly after the words *sport* and *numerous*.

Example 1: *There are many advantages to running as a sport, of which the top advantages are:*

Example 2: *The school supplies necessary were numerous, of which a few are:*

Parallelism

Often clues to the best answer are given within the text, if you know where to look for them. The correct answer will often be parallel in grammar type, punctuation, format, and tense as the rest of the sentence.

Grammar Type

If a series of nouns is given, then make sure your choice is a noun. If those nouns are plural, then ensure that your choice is plural.

Example: *schools, politics, and governments*

If a series of verbs is given, then make sure your choice is a verb.

Example: *eat, sleep, and drink*

If a series of infinitives is given, then make sure your choice is an infinitive.

Example: *to trust, to honor, and to obey*

If a series of phrases is given, then make sure your choice is a similar phrase.

Example: *of controlling, of policing, and of maintaining*

Punctuation

If a section of text has an opening dash, parentheses, or comma at the beginning of a phrase, then you can be sure there should be a matching closing dash, parentheses, or comma at the end of the phrase. If items in a series all have commas between them, then any additional items in that series will also gain commas. Do not alternate punctuation. If a dash is at the beginning of a statement, then do not put a parenthesis at the ending of the statement.

Tense

Items in a series will also have the same tense.

If past tense is being used for the other items in the series, then maintain the same past tense for your response.

Example: *sailed, flew, and raced*

If present participle tense is being used for the other items in the series, then maintain the same present participle tense for your response.

Example: *sailing, flying, and racing*

In order to test the tense of a verb, you can put it into a sentence with yourself as the subject. *I sailed the boat. I flew the plane. I raced the car.* These all fit into similar sentence structures and are in fact the same tense.

Added Phrases

Any sentence or phrase added to a paragraph must maintain the same train of thought. This is particularly true when the word *and* is used. The word *and* joins two comments of like nature.

Example: *These men were tough. They were accustomed to a hard life, and could watch a man die without blinking.*

If an added phrase does not maintain a consistent train of thought, it will be set out with a word such as *but, however,* or *although*. The new phrase would then be inconsistent to the train of thought and would offer a contrast.

Example: *These men were tough. They were accustomed to a hard life, but to watch a man die would cause them to faint.*

A tough man accustomed to a hard life is not expected to faint. Therefore the statements are contrasting and must have a contrasting transitional word, such as *but*.

Word Confusion

Contractions
All contractions, such as *they're, it's,* and *who's* are actually two words joined together by the use of an apostrophe to replace a missing letter or letters. Whenever a contraction is encountered, it can be broken down into the two distinct words that make it up.

Example: *I wouldn't eat in the cafeteria.* = *I would not eat in the cafeteria.*

The apostrophe in the contraction is always located where the missing letter or letters should be. In the examples below, the apostrophe replaces the *o* in the word *not*. The contraction *doesn't* actually stands for the two words *does not*.

Incorrect Example: *He does'nt live here.*

Correct Example: *He doesn't live here.*

Whenever there is a contraction in an answer choice, it can always be replaced by the two words that make the contraction up. If necessary, scratch through the contractions in the choices, and replace them with the two words that make up the contraction. Otherwise the choices may be confusing. Alternatively, while reading the answer choices to yourself, instead of reading the contractions as a contraction, read them as the two separate words that make them up. Some contractions are especially confusing.

Its/It's
It's is a contraction for the two words *it is*. Don't confuse *it's* for the possessive pronoun *its*. *It's* should only be used when the two words *it is* would make sense as a replacement. Use *its* in all other cases.

Example 1: *It's going to rain later today.* = *It is going to rain later today.*

Example 2: *The dog chewed through its rope and ran away.*

They're/Their/There
They're is a contraction for they are, and those two words should always be able to replace *they're* when it is encountered.

Example: *They're going to the movie with us.* = *They are going to the movie with us.*

Their is an adjective used to show ownership.

Example 1: *Their car is a red convertible.*

Example 2: *The students from each school sat in their own stands.*

There should be used in all other cases.

Example 1: *There exists an answer to every question.*

Example 2: *The man was over there.*

Who's/Whose
Who's is a contraction for *who is*, and those two words should always be able to replace *who's* when it is encountered.

Example: *Who's going with me?* = *Who is going with me?*

Whose indicates possession, and would be used in all other cases.

Example: *Whose car is this?*

Their/His
Their is a plural possessive pronoun, referring to multiple people or objects.

Example: *The men went to their cars.*

His is a singular possessive, referring to an individual person.

Example: *Each man went to his car.*

That/Who
That may be used to refer to either persons or things.

Example 1: *Is this the only book that Louis L'Amour wrote?*

Example 2: *Is Louis L'Amour the author that [or who] wrote* The Shadow Riders?

Who should only be used to refer to persons or animals.

Example: *Mozart was the composer who wrote those operas.*

Who/Whom or Whoever/Whomever
Who/whom will be encountered in two forms, as an interrogative pronoun in a question, or as a relative pronoun not in a question.

1. Interrogative pronoun in a question.

If the answer to the question would include the pronouns *he, she, we,* or *they*, then *who* is correct.

Example: *Who threw the ball? He threw the ball.*

If the answer to the question would include the pronouns *him, her, us,* or *them*, then *whom* is correct.

Example: *With whom did you play baseball? I played baseball with him.*

2. Relative pronoun NOT in a question.

If *who/whom* is followed by a verb you should usually use *who*.

Example: *Peter Jackson was an obscure director who became a celebrity overnight.*

If *who/whom* is followed by a noun, you should usually use "whom".

Example: *Bob, whom we follow throughout his career, rose swiftly up the ladder of success.*

However, beware of the insertion of phrases or expressions immediately following the use of *who/whom*. Sometimes, the phrase can be skipped without the sentence losing its meaning.

Example: *This is the woman who, we believe, will win the race.*

To determine the proper selection of *who/whom*, skip the phrase *we believe*. Thus, *who* would come before *will win,* a verb, making the choice of *who* correct.

In other cases, the sentence should be rephrased in order to make the right decision.

Example: *I can't remember who the author of* War and Peace *is*.

To determine the proper selection of *who/whom*, rephrase the sentence to state *I can't remember who is the author of* War and Peace.

Correct Pronoun Usage in Combinations
To determine the correct pronoun form in a compound subject, try each subject separately with the verb, adapting the form as necessary. Your ear will tell you which form is correct.

Example: *Bob and (I, me) will be going.*

Rephrase the sentence as two sentences, using each subject individually. *Bob will be going. I will be going.* This makes it clear, as *me will be going* does not make sense.

When a pronoun is used with a noun immediately following (as in *we boys)*, say the sentence without the added noun. Your ear will tell you the correct pronoun form.

Example: *(We/Us) boys played football last year.*

Rephrase the sentence as two sentences, without the noun. *We played football last year. Us played football last year.* Clearly *we played football last year* makes more sense.

Commas

Flow
Commas break the flow of text. To test whether they are necessary, while reading, pause for a moment at each comma. If the pauses seem natural, then the commas are correct. If they are not, then the commas are not correct.

Nonessential Clauses and Phrases
A comma should be used to set off nonessential clauses and nonessential participial phrases from the rest of the sentence. To determine if a clause is essential, remove it from the sentence. If the removal of the clause would alter the meaning of the sentence, then it is essential. Otherwise, it is nonessential.

Example: *John Smith, who was a disciple of Andrew Collins, was a noted archeologist.*

In the example above, the sentence describes John Smith's fame in archeology. The fact that he was a disciple of Andrew Collins is not necessary to that meaning. Therefore, separating it from the rest of the sentence with commas is correct.

Do not use a comma if the clause or phrase is essential to the meaning of the sentence.

Example: *Anyone who appreciates obscure French poetry will enjoy reading the book.*

If the phrase *who appreciates obscure French poetry* is removed, the sentence would indicate that anyone would enjoy reading the book, not just those with an appreciation for obscure French poetry. However, the sentence implies that the book may not be for everyone, so the phrase is essential.

Another, perhaps easier, way to determine if the clause is essential is to see if it has a comma at its beginning or end. Consistent, parallel punctuation must be used, and so if you can determine a comma exists at one side of the clause, then you can be certain that a comma should exist on the opposite side.

<u>Subjects and Verbs</u>
Subjects and verbs must not be separated by commas. However, a pair of commas setting off a nonessential phrase is allowed.

Example: *The office, which closed today for the festival, was open on Thursday.*

The verb is *was*, while *office* is the subject. The comma pair between them sets off a nonessential phrase, *which closed today for the festival*. A single comma between them would not be appropriate.

If you are trying to find the subject, first find the verb and use it to fill in the blank in the following sentence. Who or what _____?

Example: *The boy on the bicycle raced down the hill.*

The verb is *raced*. If you can find *raced* and identify it as the verb, ask yourself, *Who or what raced down the hill?* The answer to that question is the subject. In this case it's *boy*.

<u>Independent Clauses</u>
Use a comma before the words *and, but, or, nor, for,* or *yet* when they join independent clauses. To determine if two clauses are independent, remove the word that joins them. If each separate clause is capable of being a complete sentence by itself, then they are independent and need a comma between them.

Example: He ran down the street, and then he ran over the bridge.

He ran down the street. Then he ran over the bridge. Each clause is capable of being a complete sentence. Therefore a comma must be used along with the word *and* to join the two clauses together.

If one or more of the clauses would be a fragment on its own, then it must be joined to another clause and no comma is needed between them.

Example: *He ran down the street and over the bridge.*

He ran down the street. Over the bridge. The phrase *over the bridge* is a sentence fragment and is not capable of existing on its own. No comma is necessary to join it with *He ran down the street*.

Note that this does not cover the use of *and* when separating items in a series, such as *red, white, and blue*. In these cases a comma is not always necessary between the last two items in the series, but in general it is best to use one.

Parenthetical Expressions
Commas should separate parenthetical expressions such as the following: *after all, by the way, for example, in fact, on the other hand.*

Example: *By the way, she is in my biology class.*

If the parenthetical expression is in the middle of the sentence, a comma should be placed before and after it.

Example: *She is, after all, in my biology class.*

However, these expressions are not always used parenthetically. In these cases, commas are not used. To determine if an expression is parenthetical, see if it would need a pause if you were reading the text. If it does, then it is parenthetical and needs commas.

Example: *You can tell by the way she plays the violin that she enjoys its music.*

No pause is necessary in reading that example sentence. Therefore, the phrase *by the way* does not need commas around it.

Sentence Beginnings
Use a comma after words such as *so, well, yes, no,* and *why* when they begin a sentence.

Example 1: *So, you were there when they visited.*
Example 2: *Well, I really haven't thought about it.*
Example 3: *Yes, I heard your question.*
Example 4: *No, I don't think I'll go to the movie.*
Example 5: *Why, I can't imagine where I left my keys.*

Hyphens

Hyphenate a compound adjective that is directly before the noun it describes.

Example 1: *He was the best-known kid in the school.*
Example 2: *The shot came from that grass-covered hill.*
Example 3: *The well-drained fields were dry soon after the rain.*

Semicolons

Period Replacement
A semicolon is often described as either a weak period or a strong comma. Semicolons should separate independent clauses that could stand alone as separate sentences. To test where a semicolon should go, replace it with a period in your mind. If the two independent clauses would seem normal with the period, then the semicolon is in the right place.

Example: *The rain had finally stopped; a few rays of sunshine were pushing their way through the clouds.*

The rain had finally stopped. A few rays of sunshine were pushing their way through the clouds. These two sentences can exist independently with a period between them. Because they are also closely related in thought, a semicolon is a good choice to combine them.

Related/Unrelated
A semicolon should only join clauses that are closely related in thought.

Example: *The lasagna is delicious; I'll have another piece.*

In this example, the two clauses are closely related in thought. Therefore, a semicolon should join them.

Do not use a semicolon if the clauses are unrelated in thought.

Example: *For Steve, oil painting was a difficult medium to master. He had enjoyed taking photographs when he was younger.*

In this example, the two sentences would be unrelated clauses, so a semicolon should not join them.

Comparative Methods of Joining Clauses
Use a semicolon between independent clauses not joined by *and, but, for, or, nor, yet, so, since, therefore*. Semicolons should rarely be next to these words, as they are used in place of a comma combined with one of these words.

Example 1: *He had the gun; it hung from a holster at his side.*

In the example above, no *and* or comma is necessary.

Example 2: *He had the gun, and it hung from a holster at his side.*

In the example above, the comma combines with the word *and* to join the two independent clauses.

Transitions
When a semicolon is next to a transition word, such as *however*, it comes before the word.

Example: *The man in the red shirt stood next to her; however, he did not know her name.*

If these two clauses were separated with a period, the period would go before the word *however*, creating the following two sentences: *The man in the red shirt stood next to her. However, he did not know her name.* The semicolon can function as a weak period and join the two clauses by replacing the period.

Items in a Series
Semicolons are used to separate 3 or more items in a series that have a comma internally.

Example: *The club president appointed the following to chair the various committees: John Smith, planning; Jessica Graham, membership; Paul Randolph, financial; and Jerry Short, legal.*

Parentheses

Years
Parentheses should be used around years.

Example: *The presidency of Franklin Delano Roosevelt (1932-1945) was the longest one in American history.*

Nonessential Information
Parentheses can be used around information that is added to a sentence but is not essential. Commas or dashes could also be used around these nonessential phrases.

Example: *George Eliot (whose real name was Mary Ann Evans) wrote poems and several well-known novels.*

Items in a Series
A colon should precede a list of items in which you could logically insert the word *namely* after it.

Example: *The syllabus stated that each student would need the following: a sketch pad, a set of paint brushes, an easel, a pencil, and a box of crayons.*

When the list immediately follows a verb or preposition, do not use a colon.

Example 1: *The emergency kit included safety flares, jumper cables, and a flashlight.*

Example 2: *Each student taking the test was provided with two sharpened pencils, paper, a calculator, and a ruler.*

Note that the insertion of the word *namely* would be awkward in the above two examples.

Independent Clauses
Use a colon between independent clauses when the second clause explains or restates the idea of the first.

Example: *Benjamin Franklin had many talents: he was an inventor, a writer, a politician, and a philosopher.*

Apostrophes

If a noun is plural and ends in an *s*, the possessive apostrophe would come after the word, without the addition of another *s*.

Example: *The students' hats were wet from the rain.*

In the example above, there are multiple students, all of whom have wet hats.

If a noun is plural and does not end in an *s*, the possessive apostrophe would come after the word, with the addition of an *s*.

Example: *The mice's feet were wet from the rain.*

If a noun is singular, the possessive apostrophe is followed by an *s*.

Example: *The student's hat was wet from the rain.*

In the example above, there is only one student, whose hat is wet.

The Math Test

Pre-Algebra and Algebra

Numbers and Their Classifications

Numbers are the basic building blocks of mathematics. Specific features of numbers are identified by the following terms:
- Integers – The set of whole positive and negative numbers, including zero. Integers do not include fractions ($\frac{1}{3}$), decimals (0.56), or mixed numbers ($7\frac{3}{4}$).
- Prime number – A whole number greater than 1 that has only two factors, itself and 1; that is, a number that can be divided evenly only by 1 and itself.
- Composite number – A whole number greater than 1 that has more than two different factors; in other words, any whole number that is not a prime number. For example: The composite number 8 has the factors of 1, 2, 4, and 8.
- Even number – Any integer that can be divided by 2 without leaving a remainder. For example: 2, 4, 6, 8, and so on.
- Odd number – Any integer that cannot be divided evenly by 2. For example: 3, 5, 7, 9, and so on.
- Decimal number – a number that uses a decimal point to show the part of the number that is less than one. Example: 1.234.
- Decimal point – a symbol used to separate the ones place from the tenths place in decimals or dollars from cents in currency.
- Decimal place – the position of a number to the right of the decimal point. In the decimal 0.123, the 1 is in the first place to the right of the decimal point, indicating tenths; the 2 is in the second place, indicating hundredths; and the 3 is in the third place, indicating thousandths.

The decimal, or base 10, system is a number system that uses ten different digits (0, 1, 2, 3, 4, 5, 6, 7, 8, 9). An example of a number system that uses something other than ten digits is the binary, or base 2, number system, used by computers, which uses only the numbers 0 and 1. It is thought that the decimal system originated because people had only their 10 fingers for counting.

Rational, irrational, and real numbers can be described as follows:
- Rational numbers include all integers, decimals, and fractions. Any terminating or repeating decimal number is a rational number.
- Irrational numbers cannot be written as fractions or decimals because the number of decimal places is infinite and there is no recurring pattern of digits within the number. For example, pi (π) begins with 3.141592 and continues without terminating or repeating, so pi is an irrational number.
- Real numbers are the set of all rational and irrational numbers.

Operations

There are four basic mathematical operations:
- Addition increases the value of one quantity by the value of another quantity. *Example*: $2 + 4 = 6; 8 + 9 = 17$. The result is called the sum. With addition, the order does not matter. $4 + 2 = 2 + 4$.
- Subtraction is the opposite operation to addition; it decreases the value of one quantity by the value of another quantity. *Example*: $6 - 4 = 2; 17 - 8 = 9$. The result is called the difference. Note that with subtraction, the order does matter. $6 - 4 \neq 4 - 6$.
- Multiplication can be thought of as repeated addition. One number tells how many times to add the other number to itself. *Example*: 3×2 (three times two) $= 2 + 2 + 2 = 6$. With multiplication, the order does not matter. $2 \times 3 = 3 \times 2$ or $3 + 3 = 2 + 2 + 2$.
- Division is the opposite operation to multiplication; one number tells us how many parts to divide the other number into. *Example*: $20 \div 4 = 5$; if 20 is split into 4 equal parts, each part is 5. With division, the order of the numbers does matter. $20 \div 4 \neq 4 \div 20$.

An exponent is a superscript number placed next to another number at the top right. It indicates how many times the base number is to be multiplied by itself. Exponents provide a shorthand way to write what would be a longer mathematical expression. *Example*: $a^2 = a \times a$; $2^4 = 2 \times 2 \times 2 \times 2$. A number with an exponent of 2 is said to be "squared," while a number with an exponent of 3 is said to be "cubed."

The value of a number raised to an exponent is called its power. So, 8^4 is read as "8 to the 4th power," or "8 raised to the power of 4." A negative exponent is the same as the reciprocal of a positive exponent. *Example*: $a^{-2} = \frac{1}{a^2}$.

Parentheses are used to designate which operations should be done first when there are multiple operations. *Example*: $4 - (2 + 1) = 1$; the parentheses tell us that we must add 2 and 1, and then subtract the sum from 4, rather than subtracting 2 from 4 and then adding 1 (this would give us an answer of 3).

Order of Operations is a set of rules that dictates the order in which we must perform each operation in an expression so that we will evaluate it accurately. If we have an expression that includes multiple different operations, Order of Operations tells us which operations to do first. The most common mnemonic for Order of Operations is PEMDAS, or "Please Excuse My Dear Aunt Sally." PEMDAS stands for Parentheses, Exponents, Multiplication, Division, Addition, Subtraction. It is important to understand that multiplication and division have equal precedence, as do addition and subtraction, so those pairs of operations are simply worked from left to right in order.

Example: Evaluate the expression $5 + 20 \div 4 \times (2 + 3)^2 - 6$ using the correct order of operations.
- P: Perform the operations inside the parentheses, $(2 + 3) = 5$.
- E: Simplify the exponents, $(5)^2 = 25$.
- The equation now looks like this: $5 + 20 \div 4 \times 25 - 6$.
- MD: Perform multiplication and division from left to right, $20 \div 4 = 5$; then $5 \times 25 = 125$.
- The equation now looks like this: $5 + 125 - 6$.
- AS: Perform addition and subtraction from left to right, $5 + 125 = 130$; then $130 - 6 = 124$.

The laws of exponents are as follows:
1) Any number to the power of 1 is equal to itself: $a^1 = a$.
2) The number 1 raised to any power is equal to 1: $1^n = 1$.
3) Any number raised to the power of 0 is equal to 1: $a^0 = 1$.
4) Add exponents to multiply powers of the same base number: $a^n \times a^m = a^{n+m}$.
5) Subtract exponents to divide powers of the same number; that is $a^n \div a^m = a^{n-m}$.
6) Multiply exponents to raise a power to a power: $(a^n)^m = a^{n \times m}$.
7) If multiplied or divided numbers inside parentheses are collectively raised to a power, this is the same as each individual term being raised to that power: $(a \times b)^n = a^n \times b^n$; $(a \div b)^n = a^n \div b^n$.

Note: Exponents do not have to be integers. Fractional or decimal exponents follow all the rules above as well. *Example*: $5^{\frac{1}{4}} \times 5^{\frac{3}{4}} = 5^{\frac{1}{4}+\frac{3}{4}} = 5^1 = 5$.

A root, such as a square root, is another way of writing a fractional exponent. Instead of using a superscript, roots use the radical symbol ($\sqrt{}$) to indicate the operation. A radical will have a number underneath the bar, and may sometimes have a number in the upper left: $\sqrt[n]{a}$, read as "the nth root of a." The relationship between radical notation and exponent notation can be described by this equation: $\sqrt[n]{a} = a^{\frac{1}{n}}$. The two special cases of $n = 2$ and $n = 3$ are called square roots and cube roots. If there is no number to the upper left, it is understood to be a square root ($n = 2$). Nearly all of the roots you encounter will be square roots. A square root is the same as a number raised to the one-half power. When we say that a is the square root of b ($a = \sqrt{b}$), we mean that a multiplied by itself equals b: ($a \times a = b$).

A perfect square is a number that has an integer for its square root. There are 10 perfect squares from 1 to 100: 1, 4, 9, 16, 25, 36, 49, 64, 81, 100 (the squares of integers 1 through 10).

Scientific notation is a way of writing large numbers in a shorter form. The form $a \times 10^n$ is used in scientific notation, where a is greater than or equal to 1, but less than 10, and n is the number of places the decimal must move to get from the original number to a. *Example*: The number 230,400,000 is cumbersome to write. To write the value in scientific notation, place a decimal point between the first and second numbers, and include all digits through the last non-zero digit ($a = 2.304$). To find the appropriate power of 10, count the number of places the decimal point had to move ($n = 8$). The number is positive if the decimal moved to the left, and negative if it moved to the right. We can then write 230,400,000 as 2.304×10^8. If we look instead at the number 0.00002304, we have the same value for a, but this time the decimal moved 5 places to the right ($n = -5$). Thus, 0.00002304 can be written as 2.304×10^{-5}. Using this notation makes it simple to compare very large or very small numbers. By comparing exponents, it is easy to see that 3.28×10^4 is smaller than 1.51×10^5, because 4 is less than 5.

Positive & Negative Numbers

A precursor to working with negative numbers is understanding what absolute values are. A number's absolute value is simply the distance away from zero a number is on the number line. The absolute value of a number is always positive and is written $|x|$.

When adding signed numbers, if the signs are the same simply add the absolute values of the addends and apply the original sign to the sum. For example, $(+4) + (+8) = +12$ and $(-4) + (-8) = -12$. When the original signs are different, take the absolute values of the addends and subtract the smaller value from the larger value, then apply the original sign of the larger value to the difference. For instance, $(+4) + (-8) = -4$ and $(-4) + (+8) = +4$.

For subtracting signed numbers, change the sign of the number after the minus symbol and then follow the same rules used for addition. For example, $(+4) - (+8) = (+4) + (-8) = -4$.

If the signs are the same the product is positive when multiplying signed numbers. For example, $(+4) \times (+8) = +32$ and $(-4) \times (-8) = +32$. If the signs are opposite, the product is negative. For example, $(+4) \times (-8) = -32$ and $(-4) \times (+8) = -32$. When more than two factors are multiplied together, the sign of the product is determined by how many negative factors are present. If there are an odd number of negative factors then the product is negative, whereas an even number of negative factors indicates a positive product. For instance, $(+4) \times (-8) \times (-2) = +64$ and $(-4) \times (-8) \times (-2) = -64$.

The rules for dividing signed numbers are similar to multiplying signed numbers. If the dividend and divisor have the same sign, the quotient is positive. If the dividend and divisor have opposite signs, the quotient is negative. For example, $(-4) \div (+8) = -0.5$.

Factors and Multiples

Factors are numbers that are multiplied together to obtain a product. For example, in the equation $2 \times 3 = 6$, the numbers 2 and 3 are factors. A prime number has only two factors (1 and itself), but other numbers can have many factors.

A common factor is a number that divides exactly into two or more other numbers. For example, the factors of 12 are 1, 2, 3, 4, 6, and 12, while the factors of 15 are 1, 3, 5, and 15. The common factors of 12 and 15 are 1 and 3. A prime factor is also a prime number. Therefore, the prime factors of 12 are 2 and 3. For 15, the prime factors are 3 and 5.

The greatest common factor (GCF) is the largest number that is a factor of two or more numbers. For example, the factors of 15 are 1, 3, 5, and 15; the factors of 35 are 1, 5, 7, and 35. Therefore, the greatest common factor of 15 and 35 is 5.

The least common multiple (LCM) is the smallest number that is a multiple of two or more numbers. For example, the multiples of 3 include 3, 6, 9, 12, 15, etc.; the multiples of 5 include 5, 10, 15, 20, etc. Therefore, the least common multiple of 3 and 5 is 15.

Fractions, Percentages, and Related Concepts

A fraction is a number that is expressed as one integer written above another integer, with a dividing line between them ($\frac{x}{y}$). It represents the quotient of the two numbers "x divided by y." It can also be thought of as x out of y equal parts.

The top number of a fraction is called the numerator, and it represents the number of parts under consideration. The 1 in $\frac{1}{4}$ means that 1 part out of the whole is being considered in the calculation. The bottom number of a fraction is called the denominator, and it represents the total number of equal parts. The 4 in $\frac{1}{4}$ means that the whole consists of 4 equal parts. A fraction cannot have a denominator of zero; this is referred to as "undefined."

Fractions can be manipulated, without changing the value of the fraction, by multiplying or dividing (but not adding or subtracting) both the numerator and denominator by the same number. If you divide both numbers by a common factor, you are reducing or simplifying the fraction. Two fractions that have the same value, but are expressed differently are known as equivalent fractions. For example, $\frac{2}{10}, \frac{3}{15}, \frac{4}{20}$, and $\frac{5}{25}$ are all equivalent fractions. They can also all be reduced or simplified to $\frac{1}{5}$.

When two fractions are manipulated so that they have the same denominator, this is known as finding a common denominator. The number chosen to be that common denominator should be the least common multiple of the two original denominators. *Example:* $\frac{3}{4}$ and $\frac{5}{6}$; the least common multiple of 4 and 6 is 12. Manipulating to achieve the common denominator: $\frac{3}{4} = \frac{9}{12}; \frac{5}{6} = \frac{10}{12}$.

If two fractions have a common denominator, they can be added or subtracted simply by adding or subtracting the two numerators and retaining the same denominator. *Example:* $\frac{1}{2} + \frac{1}{4} = \frac{2}{4} + \frac{1}{4} = \frac{3}{4}$. If the two fractions do not already have the same denominator, one or both of them must be manipulated to achieve a common denominator before they can be added or subtracted.

Two fractions can be multiplied by multiplying the two numerators to find the new numerator and the two denominators to find the new denominator. *Example:* $\frac{1}{3} \times \frac{2}{3} = \frac{1 \times 2}{3 \times 3} = \frac{2}{9}$.

Two fractions can be divided by flipping the numerator and denominator of the second fraction and then proceeding as though it were a multiplication. *Example:* $\frac{2}{3} \div \frac{3}{4} = \frac{2}{3} \times \frac{4}{3} = \frac{8}{9}$.

A fraction whose denominator is greater than its numerator is known as a proper fraction, while a fraction whose numerator is greater than its denominator is known as an improper fraction. Proper fractions have values less than one and improper fractions have values greater than one.

A mixed number is a number that contains both an integer and a fraction. Any improper fraction can be rewritten as a mixed number. *Example:* $\frac{8}{3} = \frac{6}{3} + \frac{2}{3} = 2 + \frac{2}{3} = 2\frac{2}{3}$. Similarly, any mixed number can be rewritten as an improper fraction. *Example:* $1\frac{3}{5} = 1 + \frac{3}{5} = \frac{5}{5} + \frac{3}{5} = \frac{8}{5}$.

Percentages can be thought of as fractions that are based on a whole of 100; that is, one whole is equal to 100%. The word percent means "per hundred." Fractions can be expressed as percents by finding equivalent fractions with a denomination of 100. *Example:* $\frac{7}{10} = \frac{70}{100} = 70\%$; $\frac{1}{4} = \frac{25}{100} = 25\%$.

To express a percentage as a fraction, divide the percentage number by 100 and reduce the fraction to its simplest possible terms. *Example:* $60\% = \frac{60}{100} = \frac{3}{5}$; $96\% = \frac{96}{100} = \frac{24}{25}$.

Converting decimals to percentages and percentages to decimals is as simple as moving the decimal point. To convert from a decimal to a percent, move the decimal point two places to the right. To convert from a percent to a decimal, move it two places to the left. *Example:* 0.23 = 23%; 5.34 = 534%; 0.007 = 0.7%; 700% = 7.00; 86% = 0.86; 0.15% = 0.0015.

It may be helpful to remember that the percentage number will always be larger than the equivalent decimal number.

A percentage problem can be presented three main ways: (1) Find what percentage of some number another number is. *Example:* What percentage of 40 is 8? (2) Find what number is some percentage of a given number. *Example:* What number is 20% of 40? (3) Find what number another number is a given percentage of. *Example:* What number is 8 20% of? The three components in all of these cases are the same: a whole (*W*), a part (*P*), and a percentage (%). These are related by the equation: $P = W \times \%$. This is the form of the equation you would use to solve problems of type (2). To solve types (1) and (3), you would use these two forms: $\% = \frac{P}{W}$ and $W = \frac{P}{\%}$.

The thing that frequently makes percentage problems difficult is that they are most often also word problems, so a large part of solving them is figuring out which quantities are what. Here's an example: *In a school cafeteria, 7 students choose pizza, 9 choose hamburgers, and 4 choose tacos. Find the percentage that chooses tacos.* To find the whole, you must first add all of the parts: 7 + 9 + 4 = 20. The percentage can then be found by dividing the part by the whole(% = $\frac{P}{W}$): $\frac{4}{20} = \frac{20}{100} = 20\%$.

A ratio is a comparison of two quantities in a particular order. *Example*: If there are 14 computers in a lab, and the class has 20 students, there is a student to computer ratio of 20 to 14, commonly written as 20:14. Ratios are normally reduced to their smallest whole number representation, so 20:14 would be reduced to 10:7 by dividing both sides by 2.

A proportion is a relationship between two quantities that dictates how one changes when the other changes. A direct proportion describes a relationship in which a quantity increases by a set amount for every increase in the other quantity, or decreases by that same amount for every decrease in the other quantity. *Example*: Assuming a constant driving speed, the time required for a car trip increases as the distance of the trip increases. The distance to be traveled and the time required to travel are directly proportional.

Inverse proportion is a relationship in which an increase in one quantity is accompanied by a decrease in the other, or vice versa. *Example*: the time required for a car trip decreases as the speed increases, and increases as the speed decreases, so the time required is inversely proportional to the speed of the car.

Equations and Graphing

When algebraic functions and equations are shown graphically, they are usually shown on a *Cartesian Coordinate Plane*. The Cartesian coordinate plane consists of two number lines placed perpendicular to each other, and intersecting at the zero point, also known as the origin. The horizontal number line is known as the *x*-axis, with positive values to the right of the origin, and negative values to the left of the origin. The vertical number line is known as the *y*-axis, with positive values above the origin, and negative values below the origin. Any point on the plane can be identified by an ordered pair in the form (*x,y*), called coordinates. The *x*-value of the coordinate is called the abscissa, and the *y*-value of the coordinate is called the ordinate. The two number lines divide the plane into four quadrants: I, II, III, and IV.

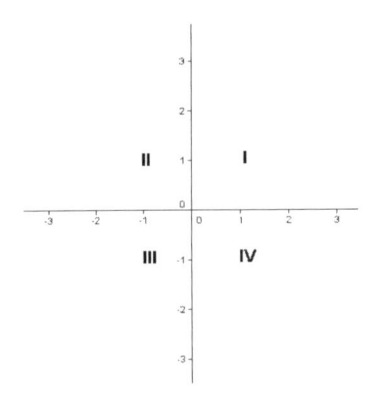

Before learning the different forms equations can be written in, it is important to understand some terminology. A ratio of the change in the vertical distance to the change in horizontal distance is called the *Slope*. On a graph with two points, (x_1, y_1) and (x_2, y_2), the slope is represented by the formula $= \frac{y_2 - y_1}{x_2 - x_1}$; $x_1 \neq x_2$. If the value of the slope is positive, the line slopes upward from left to right. If the value of the slope is negative, the line slopes downward from left to right. If the *y*-coordinates are the same for both points, the slope is 0 and the line is a *Horizontal Line*. If the *x*-

coordinates are the same for both points, there is no slope and the line is a *Vertical Line*. Two or more lines that have equal slopes are *Parallel Lines*. *Perpendicular Lines* have slopes that are negative reciprocals of each other, such as $\frac{a}{b}$ and $\frac{-b}{a}$.

Equations are made up of monomials and polynomials. A *Monomial* is a single variable or product of constants and variables, such as x, $2x$, or $\frac{2}{x}$. There will never be addition or subtraction symbols in a monomial. Like monomials have like variables, but they may have different coefficients. *Polynomials* are algebraic expressions which use addition and subtraction to combine two or more monomials. Two terms make a binomial; three terms make a trinomial; etc.. The *Degree of a Monomial* is the sum of the exponents of the variables. The *Degree of a Polynomial* is the highest degree of any individual term.

As mentioned previously, equations can be written many ways. Below is a list of the many forms equations can take.
- *Standard Form*: $Ax + By = C$; the slope is $\frac{-A}{B}$ and the y-intercept is $\frac{C}{B}$
- *Slope Intercept Form*: $y = mx + b$, where m is the slope and b is the y-intercept
- *Point-Slope Form*: $y - y_1 = m(x - x_1)$, where m is the slope and (x_1, y_1) is a point on the line
- *Two-Point Form*: $\frac{y-y_1}{x-x_1} = \frac{y_2-y_1}{x_2-x_1}$, where (x_1, y_1) and (x_2, y_2) are two points on the given line
- *Intercept Form*: $\frac{x}{x_1} + \frac{y}{y_1} = 1$, where $(x_1, 0)$ is the point at which a line intersects the x-axis, and $(0, y_1)$ is the point at which the same line intersects the y-axis

Equations can also be written as $ax + b = 0$, where $a \neq 0$. These are referred to as *One Variable Linear Equations*. A solution to such an equation is called a *Root*. In the case where we have the equation $5x + 10 = 0$, if we solve for x we get a solution of $x = -2$. In other words, the root of the equation is -2. This is found by first subtracting 10 from both sides, which gives $5x = -10$. Next, simply divide both sides by the coefficient of the variable, in this case 5, to get $x = -2$. This can be checked by plugging -2 back into the original equation $(5)(-2) + 10 = -10 + 10 = 0$.

The *Solution Set* is the set of all solutions of an equation. In our example, the solution set would simply be -2. If there were more solutions (there usually are in multivariable equations) then they would also be included in the solution set. When an equation has no true solutions, this is referred to as an *Empty Set*. Equations with identical solution sets are *Equivalent Equations*. An *Identity* is a term whose value or determinant is equal to 1.

Other Important Concepts

Commonly in algebra and other upper-level fields of math you find yourself working with mathematical expressions that do not equal each other. The statement comparing such expressions with symbols such as < (less than) or > (greater than) is called an *Inequality*. An example of an inequality is $7x > 5$. To solve for x, simply divide both sides by 7 and the solution is shown to be $x > \frac{5}{7}$. Graphs of the solution set of inequalities are represented on a number line. Open circles are used to show that an expression approaches a number but is never quite equal to that number.

Conditional Inequalities are those with certain values for the variable that will make the condition true and other values for the variable where the condition will be false. *Absolute Inequalities* can have any real number as the value for the variable to make the condition true, while there is no real number value for the variable that will make the condition false. Solving inequalities is done by following the same rules as for solving equations with the exception that when multiplying or dividing by a negative number the direction of the inequality sign must be flipped or reversed. *Double Inequalities* are situations where two inequality statements apply to the same variable expression. An example of this is $-c < ax + b < c$.

A *Weighted Mean*, or weighted average, is a mean that uses "weighted" values. The formula is weighted mean $= \frac{w_1x_1+w_2x_2+w_3x_3...+w_nx_n}{w_1+w_2+w_3+...+w_n}$. Weighted values, such as $w_1, w_2, w_3, ... w_n$ are assigned to each member of the set $x_1, x_2, x_3, ... x_n$. If calculating weighted mean, make sure a weight value for each member of the set is used.

Calculations Using Points

Sometimes you need to perform calculations using only points on a graph as input data. Using points, you can determine what the midpoint and distance are. If you know the equation for a line you can calculate the distance between the line and the point.

To find the *Midpoint* of two points (x_1, y_1) and (x_2, y_2), average the x-coordinates to get the x-coordinate of the midpoint, and average the y-coordinates to get the y-coordinate of the midpoint. The formula is midpoint $= \left(\frac{x_1+x_2}{2}, \frac{y_1+y_2}{2}\right)$.

The *Distance* between two points is the same as the length of the hypotenuse of a right triangle with the two given points as endpoints, and the two sides of the right triangle parallel to the x-axis and y-axis, respectively. The length of the segment parallel to the x-axis is the difference between the x-coordinates of the two points. The length of the segment parallel to the y-axis is the difference between the y-coordinates of the two points. Use the Pythagorean Theorem $a^2 + b^2 = c^2$ or $c = \sqrt{a^2 + b^2}$ to find the distance. The formula is distance $= \sqrt{(x_2 - x_1)^2 + (y_2 - y_1)^2}$.

When a line is in the format $Ax + By + C = 0$, where A, B, and C are coefficients, you can use a point (x_1, y_1) not on the line and apply the formula $d = \frac{|Ax_1+By_1+C|}{\sqrt{A^2+B^2}}$ to find the distance between the line and the point (x_1, y_1).

Systems of Equations

Systems of Equations are a set of simultaneous equations that all use the same variables. A solution to a system of equations must be true for each equation in the system. *Consistent Systems* are those with at least one solution. *Inconsistent Systems* are systems of equations that have no solution.

To solve a system of linear equations by *substitution*, start with the easier equation and solve for one of the variables. Express this variable in terms of the other variable. Substitute this expression in the other equation, and solve for the other variable. The solution should be expressed in the form (x, y). Substitute the values into both of the original equations to check your answer. Consider the following problem.

Solve the system using substitution:
$$x + 6y = 15$$
$$3x - 12y = 18$$

Solve the first equation for x:
$$x = 15 - 6y$$

Substitute this value in place of x in the second equation, and solve for y:
$$3(15 - 6y) - 12y = 18$$
$$45 - 18y - 12y = 18$$
$$30y = 27$$
$$y = \frac{27}{30} = \frac{9}{10} = 0.9$$

Plug this value for *y* back into the first equation to solve for *x*:
$$x = 15 - 6(0.9) = 15 - 5.4 = 9.6$$

Check both equations if you have time:
$$9.6 + 6(0.9) = 9.6 + 5.4 = 15$$
$$3(9.6) - 12(0.9) = 28.8 - 10.8 = 18$$

Therefore, the solution is (9.6, 0.9).

To solve a system of equations using *elimination*, begin by rewriting both equations in standard form $Ax + By = C$. Check to see if the coefficients of one pair of like variables add to zero. If not, multiply one or both of the equations by a non-zero number to make one set of like variables add to zero. Add the two equations to solve for one of the variables. Substitute this value into one of the original equations to solve for the other variable. Check your work by substituting into the other equation. Next we will solve the same problem as above, but using the addition method.

Solve the system using elimination:
$$x + 6y = 15$$
$$3x - 12y = 18$$

If we multiply the first equation by 2, we can eliminate the *y* terms:
$$2x + 12y = 30$$
$$3x - 12y = 18$$

Add the equations together and solve for *x*:
$$5x = 48$$
$$x = \frac{48}{5} = 9.6$$

Plug the value for *x* back into either of the original equations and solve for *y*:
$$9.6 + 6y = 15$$
$$y = \frac{15 - 9.6}{6} = 0.9$$

Check both equations if you have time:
$$9.6 + 6(0.9) = 9.6 + 5.4 = 15$$
$$3(9.6) - 12(0.9) = 28.8 - 10.8 = 18$$

Therefore, the solution is (9.6, 0.9).

Polynomial Algebra

To multiply two binomials, follow the *FOIL* method. FOIL stands for:
- First: Multiply the first term of each binomial
- Outer: Multiply the outer terms of each binomial
- Inner: Multiply the inner terms of each binomial
- Last: Multiply the last term of each binomial

Using FOIL, $(Ax + By)(Cx + Dy) = ACx^2 + ADxy + BCxy + BDy^2$.

To divide polynomials, begin by arranging the terms of each polynomial in order of one variable. You may arrange in ascending or descending order, but be consistent with both polynomials. To get the first term of the quotient, divide the first term of the dividend by the first term of the divisor. Multiply the first term of the quotient by the entire divisor and subtract that product from the dividend. Repeat for the second and successive terms until you either get a remainder of zero or a remainder whose degree is less than the degree of the divisor. If the quotient has a remainder, write the answer as a mixed expression in the form: quotient $+ \frac{remainder}{divisor}$.

Rational Expressions are fractions with polynomials in both the numerator and the denominator; the value of the polynomial in the denominator cannot be equal to zero. To add or subtract rational expressions, first find the common denominator, then rewrite each fraction as an equivalent fraction with the common denominator. Finally, add or subtract the numerators to get the numerator of the answer, and keep the common denominator as the denominator of the answer. When multiplying rational expressions, factor each polynomial and cancel like factors (a factor which appears in both the numerator and the denominator). Then, multiply all remaining factors in the numerator to get the numerator of the product, and multiply the remaining factors in the denominator to get the denominator of the product. Remember – cancel entire factors, not individual terms. To divide rational expressions, take the reciprocal of the divisor (the rational expression you are dividing by) and multiply by the dividend.

Below are patterns of some special products to remember: *perfect trinomial squares*, the *difference between two squares*, the *sum and difference of two cubes*, and *perfect cubes*.

- Perfect Trinomial Squares: $x^2 + 2xy + y^2 = (x + y)^2$ or $x^2 - 2xy + y^2 = (x - y)^2$
- Difference between Two Squares: $x^2 - y^2 = (x + y)(x - y)$
- Sum of Two Cubes: $x^3 + y^3 = (x + y)(x^2 - xy + y^2)$
- Note: the second factor is NOT the same as a perfect trinomial square, so do not try to factor it further.
- Difference between Two Cubes: $x^3 - y^3 = (x - y)(x^2 + xy + y^2)$
- Again, the second factor is NOT the same as a perfect trinomial square.
- Perfect Cubes: $x^3 + 3x^2y + 3xy^2 + y^3 = (x + y)^3$ and $x^3 - 3x^2y + 3xy^2 - y^3 = (x - y)^3$

In order to *factor* a polynomial, first check for a common monomial factor. When the greatest common monomial factor has been factored out, look for patterns of special products: differences of two squares, the sum or difference of two cubes for binomial factors, or perfect trinomial squares for trinomial factors. If the factor is a trinomial but not a perfect trinomial square, look for a factorable form, such as $x^2 + (a + b)x + ab = (x + a)(x + b)$ or $(ac)x^2 + (ad + bc)x + bd = (ax + b)(cx + d)$. For factors with four terms, look for groups to factor. Once you have found the factors, write the original polynomial as the product of all the factors. Make sure all of the polynomial factors are prime. Monomial factors may be prime or composite. Check your work by multiplying the factors to make sure you get the original polynomial.

Solving Quadratic Equations

The *Quadratic Formula* is used to solve quadratic equations when other methods are more difficult. To use the quadratic formula to solve a quadratic equation, begin by rewriting the equation in standard form $ax^2 + bx + c = 0$, where a, b, and c are coefficients. Once you have identified the values of the coefficients, substitute those values into the quadratic formula $x = \frac{-b \pm \sqrt{b^2 - 4ac}}{2a}$. Evaluate the equation and simplify the expression. Again, check each root by substituting into the original equation. In the quadratic formula, the portion of the formula under the radical ($b^2 - 4ac$) is called the *Discriminant*. If the discriminant is zero, there is only one root: zero. If the discriminant is positive, there are two different real roots. If the discriminant is negative, there are no real roots.

To solve a quadratic equation by *Factoring*, begin by rewriting the equation in standard form, if necessary. Factor the side with the variable then set each of the factors equal to zero and solve the resulting linear equations. Check your answers by substituting the roots you found into the original equation. If, when writing the equation in standard form, you have an equation in the form $x^2 + c = 0$ or $x^2 - c = 0$, set $x^2 = -c$ or $x^2 = c$ and take the square root of c. If $c = 0$, the only real root is zero. If c is positive, there are two real roots—the positive and negative square root values. If c is negative, there are no real roots because you cannot take the square root of a negative number.

To solve a quadratic equation by *Completing the Square*, rewrite the equation so that all terms containing the variable are on the left side of the equal sign, and all the constants are on the right side of the equal sign. Make sure the coefficient of the squared term is 1. If there is a coefficient with the squared term, divide each term on both sides of the equal side by that number. Next, work with the coefficient of the single-variable term. Square half of this coefficient, and add that value to both sides. Now you can factor the left side (the side containing the variable) as the square of a binomial. $x^2 + 2ax + a^2 = C \Rightarrow (x + a)^2 = C$, where x is the variable, and a and C are constants. Take the square root of both sides and solve for the variable. Substitute the value of the variable in the original problem to check your work.

Geometry

Geometry Concepts

Below are some terms that are commonly used in geometric studies. Most of these concepts are foundational to geometry, so understanding them is a necessary first step to studying geometry.

A point is a fixed location in space; has no size or dimensions; commonly represented by a dot.

A line is a set of points that extends infinitely in two opposite directions. It has length, but no width or depth. A line can be defined by any two distinct points that it contains. A line segment is a portion of a line that has definite endpoints. A ray is a portion of a line that extends from a single point on that line in one direction along the line. It has a definite beginning, but no ending.

A plane is a two-dimensional flat surface defined by three non-collinear points. A plane extends an infinite distance in all directions in those two dimensions. It contains an infinite number of points, parallel lines and segments, intersecting lines and segments, as well as parallel or intersecting rays. A plane will never contain a three-dimensional figure or skew lines. Two given planes will either be parallel or they will intersect to form a line. A plane may intersect a circular conic surface, such as a cone, to form conic sections, such as the parabola, hyperbola, circle or ellipse.

Perpendicular lines are lines that intersect at right angles. They are represented by the symbol ⊥. The shortest distance from a line to a point not on the line is a perpendicular segment from the point to the line.

Parallel lines are lines in the same plane that have no points in common and never meet. It is possible for lines to be in different planes, have no points in common, and never meet, but they are not parallel because they are in different planes.

A bisector is a line or line segment that divides another line segment into two equal lengths. A perpendicular bisector of a line segment is composed of points that are equidistant from the endpoints of the segment it is dividing.

Intersecting lines are lines that have exactly one point in common. Concurrent lines are multiple lines that intersect at a single point.

A transversal is a line that intersects at least two other lines, which may or may not be parallel to one another. A transversal that intersects parallel lines is a common occurrence in geometry.

Angles

An angle is formed when two lines or line segments meet at a common point. It may be a common starting point for a pair of segments or rays, or it may be the intersection of lines. Angles are represented by the symbol ∠.

The vertex is the point at which two segments or rays meet to form an angle. If the angle is formed by intersecting rays, lines, and/or line segments, the vertex is the point at which four angles are formed. The pairs of angles opposite one another are called vertical angles, and their measures are equal. In the figure below, angles ABC and DBE are congruent, as are angles ABD and CBE.

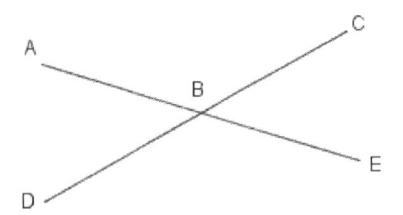

Types of angles
- An acute angle is an angle with a degree measure less than 90°.
- A right angle is an angle with a degree measure of exactly 90°.
- An obtuse angle is an angle with a degree measure greater than 90° but less than 180°.
- A straight angle is an angle with a degree measure of exactly 180°. This is also a semicircle.
- A reflex angle is an angle with a degree measure greater than 180° but less than 360°.
- A full angle is an angle with a degree measure of exactly 360°.

Two angles whose sum is exactly 90° are said to be complementary. The two angles may or may not be adjacent. In a right triangle, the two acute angles are complementary.

Two angles whose sum is exactly 180° are said to be supplementary. The two angles may or may not be adjacent. Two intersecting lines always form two pairs of supplementary angles. Adjacent supplementary angles will always form a straight line.

Two angles that have the same vertex and share a side are said to be adjacent. Vertical angles are not adjacent because they share a vertex but no common side.

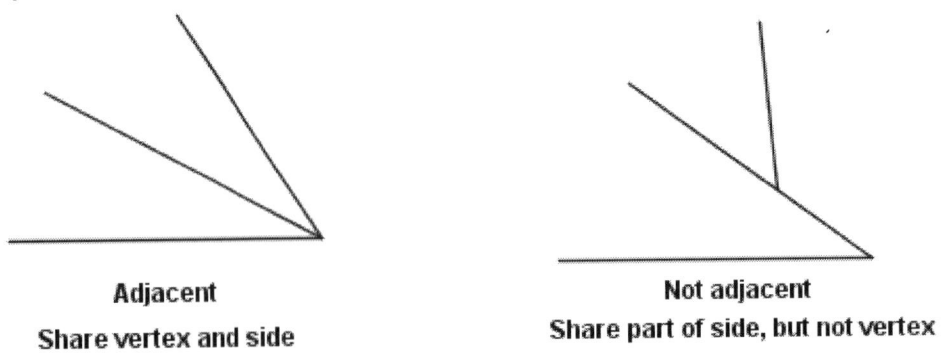

Adjacent
Share vertex and side

Not adjacent
Share part of side, but not vertex

When two parallel lines are cut by a transversal, the angles that are between the two parallel lines are interior angles. In the diagram below, angles 3, 4, 5, and 6 are interior angles.

When two parallel lines are cut by a transversal, the angles that are outside the parallel lines are exterior angles. In the following diagram, angles 1, 2, 7, and 8 are exterior angles.

When two parallel lines are cut by a transversal, the angles that are in the same position relative to the transversal and a parallel line are corresponding angles. The following diagram has four pairs of corresponding angles: angles 1 and 5; angles 2 and 6; angles 3 and 7; and angles 4 and 8. Corresponding angles formed by parallel lines are congruent.

When two parallel lines are cut by a transversal, the two interior angles that are on opposite sides of the transversal are called alternate interior angles. In the diagram below, there are two pairs of alternate interior angles: angles 3 and 6, and angles 4 and 5. Alternate interior angles formed by parallel lines are congruent.

When two parallel lines are cut by a transversal, the two exterior angles that are on opposite sides of the transversal are called alternate exterior angles. In the diagram below, there are two pairs of alternate exterior angles: angles 1 and 8, and angles 2 and 7. Alternate exterior angles formed by parallel lines are congruent.

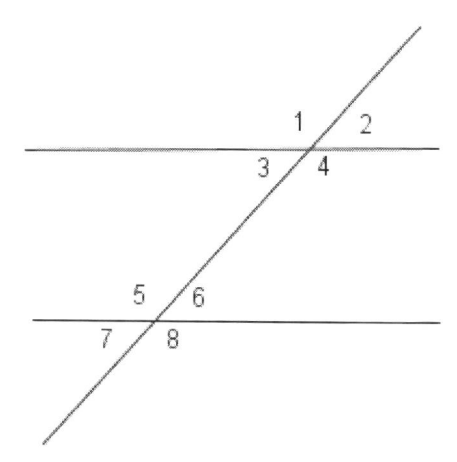

Circles

The center is the single point inside the circle that is equidistant from every point on the circle. (Point O in the diagram below.)

The radius is a line segment that joins the center of the circle and any one point on the circle. All radii of a circle are equal. (Segments OX, OY, and OZ in the diagram below.)

The diameter is a line segment that passes through the center of the circle and has both endpoints on the circle. The length of the diameter is exactly twice the length of the radius. (Segment XZ in the diagram below.)

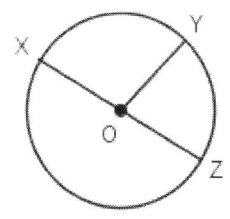

A circle is inscribed in a polygon if each of the sides of the polygon is tangent to the circle. A polygon is inscribed in a circle if each of the vertices of the polygon lies on the circle.

A circle is circumscribed about a polygon if each of the vertices of the polygon lies on the circle. A polygon is circumscribed about the circle if each of the sides of the polygon is tangent to the circle.

If one figure is inscribed in another, then the other figure is circumscribed about the first figure.

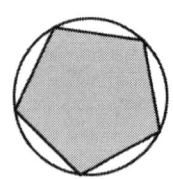

Circle circumscribed about a pentagon
Pentagon inscribed in a circle

Polygons

A polygon is a planar shape formed from line segments called sides that are joined together at points called vertices (singular: vertex). Specific polygons are named by the number of angles or sides they have. Regular polygons are polygons whose sides are all equal and whose angles are all congruent.

An interior angle is any of the angles inside a polygon where two sides meet at a vertex. The sum of the interior angles of a polygon is dependent only on the number of sides. For example, all 5-sided polygons have interior angles that sum to 540°, regardless of the particular shape.

A diagonal is a line that joins two nonconsecutive vertices of a polygon. The number of diagonals that can be drawn on an *n*-sided polygon is $d = \frac{n(n-3)}{2}$.

The following list presents several different types of polygons:
- Triangle – 3 sides
- Quadrilateral – 4 sides
- Pentagon – 5 sides
- Hexagon – 6 sides
- Heptagon – 7 sides
- Octagon – 8 sides
- Nonagon – 9 sides
- Decagon – 10 sides
- Dodecagon – 12 sides

More generally, an *n*-gon is a polygon that has *n* angles and *n* sides.

The sum of the interior angles of an *n*-sided polygon is (n – 2)180°. For example, in a triangle n = 3, so the sum of the interior angles is (3 – 2)180° = 180°. In a quadrilateral, n = 4, and the sum of the angles is (4 – 2)180° = 360°. The sum of the interior angles of a polygon is equal to the sum of the interior angles of any other polygon with the same number of sides.

Below are descriptions for several common quadrilaterals. Recall that a quadrilateral is a four-sided polygon.
- Trapezoid – quadrilateral with exactly one pair of parallel sides (opposite one another); in an isosceles trapezoid, the two non-parallel sides have equal length and both pairs of non-opposite angles are congruent
- Parallelogram – quadrilateral with two pairs of parallel sides (opposite one another), and two pairs of congruent angles (opposite one another)
- Rhombus – parallelogram with four equal sides
- Rectangle – parallelogram with four congruent angles (right angles)
- Square – parallelogram with four equal sides and four congruent angles (right angles)

Triangles

A triangle is a polygon with three sides and three angles. Triangles can be classified according to the length of their sides or magnitude of their angles.

An acute triangle is a triangle whose three angles are all less than 90°. If two of the angles are equal, the acute triangle is also an isosceles triangle. If the three angles are all equal, the acute triangle is also an equilateral triangle.

A right triangle is a triangle with exactly one angle equal to 90°. All right triangles follow the Pythagorean Theorem. A right triangle can never be acute or obtuse.

An obtuse triangle is a triangle with exactly one angle greater than 90°. The other two angles may or may not be equal. If the two remaining angles are equal, the obtuse triangle is also an isosceles triangle.

An equilateral triangle is a triangle with three congruent sides. An equilateral triangle will also have three congruent angles, each 60°. All equilateral triangles are also acute triangles.

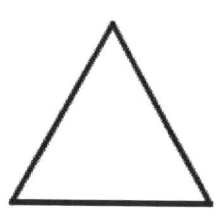

An isosceles triangle is a triangle with two congruent sides. An isosceles triangle will also have two congruent angles opposite the two congruent sides.

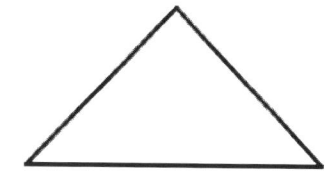

A scalene triangle is a triangle with no congruent sides. A scalene triangle will also have three angles of different measures. The angle with the largest measure is opposite the longest side, and the angle with the smallest measure is opposite the shortest side.

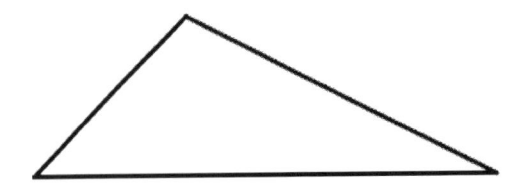

The Triangle Inequality Theorem states that the sum of the measures of any two sides of a triangle is always greater than the measure of the third side. If the sum of the measures of two sides were equal to the third side, a triangle would be impossible because the two sides would lie flat across the third side and there would be no vertex. If the sum of the measures of two of the sides was less than the third side, a closed figure would be impossible because the two shortest sides would never meet.

Similar triangles are triangles whose corresponding angles are congruent to one another. Their corresponding sides may or may not be equal, but they are proportional to one another. Since the angles in a triangle always sum to 180°, it is only necessary to determine that two pairs of corresponding angles are congruent, since in that case, the third one will also have to be.

Congruent triangles are similar triangles whose corresponding sides are all equal. Congruent triangles can be made to fit on top of one another by rotation, reflection, and/or translation. When trying to determine whether two triangles are congruent, there are several criteria that can be used.

Side-side-side (SSS): if all three sides of one triangle are equal to all three sides of another triangle, they are congruent by SSS.

Side-angle-side (SAS): if two sides and the adjoining angle in one triangle are equal to two sides and the adjoining angle of another triangle, they are congruent by SAS.

Additionally, if two triangles can be shown to be similar, then there need only be one pair of corresponding equal sides to show congruence.

One of the most important theorems in geometry is the Pythagorean Theorem. Named after the sixth-century Greek mathematician Pythagoras, this theorem states that, for a right triangle, the square of the hypotenuse (the longest side of the triangle, always opposite the right angle) is equal to the sum of the squares of the other two sides. Written symbolically, the Pythagorean Theorem can be expressed as $a^2 + b^2 = c^2$, where c is the hypotenuse and a and b are the remaining two sides.

The theorem is most commonly used to find the length of an unknown side of a right triangle, given the lengths of the other two sides. For example, given that the hypotenuse of a right triangle is 5 and one side is 3, the other side can be found using the formula: $a^2 + b^2 = c^2$, $3^2 + b^2 = 5^2$, $9 + b^2 = 25$, $b^2 = 25 - 9 = 16$, $b = \sqrt{16} = 4$.

The theorem can also be used "in reverse" to show that when the square of one side of a triangle is equal to the sum of the squares of the other two sides, the triangle must be a right triangle.

The Law of Sines states that $\frac{\sin A}{a} = \frac{\sin B}{b} = \frac{\sin C}{c}$, where A, B, and C are the angles of a triangle, and a, b, and c are the sides opposite their respective angles. This formula will work with all triangles, not just right triangles.

The Law of Cosines is given by the formula $c^2 = a^2 + b^2 - 2ab(\cos C)$, where a, b, and c are the sides of a triangle, and C is the angle opposite side c. This formula is similar to the Pythagorean Theorem, but unlike the Pythagorean Theorem, it can be used on any triangle.

Symmetry

Symmetry is a property of a shape in which the shape can be transformed by either reflection or rotation without losing its original shape and orientation. A shape that has reflection symmetry can be reflected across a line with the result being the same shape as before the reflection. A line of symmetry divides a shape into two parts, with each part being a mirror image of the other. A shape can have more than one line of symmetry. A circle, for instance, has an infinite number of lines of symmetry. When reflection symmetry is extended to three-dimensional space, it is taken to describe a solid that can be divided into mirror image parts by a plane of symmetry.

Rotational symmetry describes a shape that can be rotated about a point and achieve its original shape and orientation with less than a 360° rotation. When rotational symmetry is extended to three-dimensional space, it describes a solid that can be rotated about a line with the same conditions. Many shapes have both reflection and rotational symmetry.

Area Formulas

- Rectangle: $A = wl$, where w is the width and l is the length
- Square: $A = s^2$, where s is the length of a side.
- Triangle: $A = \frac{1}{2}bh$, where b is the length of one side (base) and h is the distance from that side to the opposite vertex measured perpendicularly (height).
- Parallelogram: $A = bh$, where b is the length of one side (base) and h is the perpendicular distance between that side and its parallel side (height).
- Trapezoid: $A = \frac{1}{2}(b_1 + b_2)h$, where b_1 and b_2 are the lengths of the two parallel sides (bases), and h is the perpendicular distance between them (height).
- Circle: $A = \pi r^2$, where π is the mathematical constant approximately equal to 3.14 and r is the distance from the center of the circle to any point on the circle (radius).

Volume Formulas

For some of these shapes, it is necessary to find the area of the base polygon before the volume of the solid can be found. This base area is represented in the volume equations as B.

- Pyramid – consists of a polygon base, and triangles connecting each side of that polygon to a vertex. The volume can be calculated as $V = \frac{1}{3}Bh$, where h is the distance between the vertex and the base polygon, measured perpendicularly.
- Prism – consists of two identical polygon bases, attached to one another on corresponding sides by parallelograms. The volume can be calculated as $V = Bh$, where h is the perpendicular distance between the two bases.
- Cube – a special type of prism in which the two bases are the same shape as the side faces. All faces are squares. The volume can be calculated as $V = s^3$, where s is the length of any side.
- Sphere – a round solid consisting of one continuous, uniformly-curved surface. The volume can be calculated as $V = \frac{4}{3}\pi r^3$, where r is the distance from the center of the sphere to any point on the surface (radius).

Trigonometry

Basic Functions

The three basic trigonometric functions are sine, cosine, and tangent.

<u>Sine</u>
The sine (sin) function has a period of 360° or 2π radians. This means that its graph makes one complete cycle every 360° or 2π. Because $\sin 0 = 0$, the graph of $y = \sin x$ begins at the origin, with the x-axis representing the angle measure, and the y-axis representing the sine of the angle. The graph of the sine function is a smooth curve that begins at the origin, peaks at the point $\left(\frac{\pi}{2}, 1\right)$, crosses the x-axis at $(\pi, 0)$, has its lowest point at $\left(\frac{3\pi}{2}, -1\right)$, and returns to the x-axis to complete one cycle at $(2\pi, 0)$.

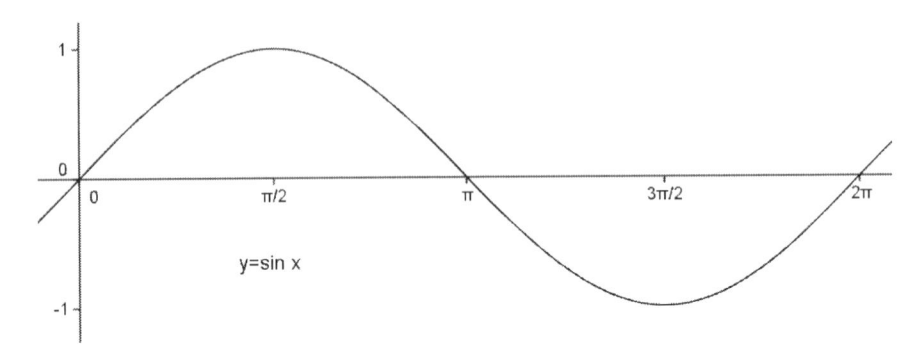

<u>Cosine</u>
The cosine (cos) function also has a period of 360° or 2π radians, which means that its graph also makes one complete cycle every 360° or 2π. Because $\cos 0° = 1$, the graph of $y = \cos x$ begins at the point $(0, 1)$, with the x-axis representing the angle measure, and the y-axis representing the cosine of the angle.

The graph of the cosine function is a smooth curve that begins at the point $(0, 1)$, crosses the x-axis at the point $\left(\frac{\pi}{2}, 0\right)$, has its lowest point at $(\pi, -1)$, crosses the x-axis again at the point $\left(\frac{3\pi}{2}, 0\right)$, and returns to a peak at the point $(2\pi, 1)$ to complete one cycle.

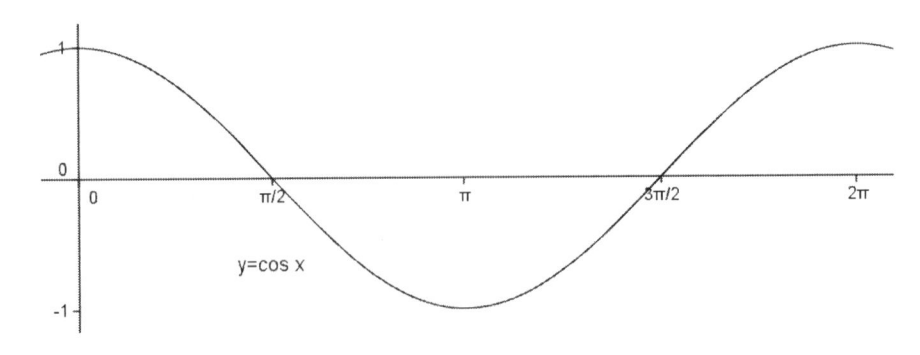

Tangent

The tangent (tan) function has a period of 180° or π radians, which means that its graph makes one complete cycle every 180° or π radians. The x-axis represents the angle measure, and the y-axis represents the tangent of the angle.

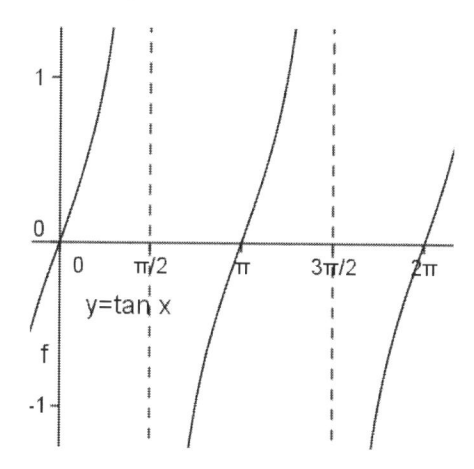

The graph of the tangent function is a series of smooth curves that cross the x-axis at every 180° or π radians and have an asymptote every $k \cdot 90°$ or $\frac{k\pi}{2}$ radians, where k is an odd integer. This can be explained by the fact that the tangent is calculated by dividing the sine by the cosine, since the cosine equals zero at those asymptote points.

Defined and Reciprocal Functions

The tangent function is defined as the ratio of the sine to the cosine:
Tangent (tan):
$$\tan x = \frac{\sin x}{\cos x}$$

To take the reciprocal of a number means to place that number as the denominator of a fraction with a numerator of 1. The reciprocal functions are thus defined quite simply.

Cosecant (csc):
$$\csc x = \frac{1}{\sin x}$$
Secant (sec):
$$\sec x = \frac{1}{\cos x}$$
Cotangent (cot):
$$\cot x = \frac{1}{\tan x}$$

It is important to know these reciprocal functions, but they are not as commonly used as the three basic functions.

Inverse Functions

Each of the trigonometric functions accepts an angular measure, either degrees or radians, and gives a numerical value as the output. The inverse functions do the opposite; they accept a numerical value and give an angular measure as the output. The inverse sine, or arcsine, commonly written as either $\sin^{-1} x$ or $\arcsin x$, gives the angle whose sine is x. Similarly:
- The inverse of cos x is written as $\cos^{-1} x$ or $\arccos x$ and means the angle whose cosine is x.
- The inverse of tan x is written as $\tan^{-1} x$ or $\arctan x$ and means the angle whose tangent is x.
- The inverse of csc x is written as $\csc^{-1} x$ or $\text{arccsc}\, x$ and means the angle whose cosecant is x.
- The inverse of sec x is written as $\sec^{-1} x$ or $\text{arcsec}\, x$ and means the angle whose secant is x.
- The inverse of cot x is written as $\cot^{-1} x$ or $\text{arccot}\, x$ and means the angle whose cotangent is x.

Important Note about Solving Trigonometric Equations
Trigonometric and algebraic equations are solved following the same rules, but while algebraic expressions have one unique solution, trigonometric equations could have multiple solutions, and you must find them all. When solving for an angle with a known trigonometric value, you must consider the sign and include all angles with that value. Your calculator will probably only give one value as an answer, typically in the following ranges:
- For the inverse sine function, $\left[-\frac{\pi}{2}, \frac{\pi}{2}\right]$ or [–90°, 90°]
- For the inverse cosine function, [0, π] or [0°, 180°]
- For the inverse tangent function, $\left[-\frac{\pi}{2}, \frac{\pi}{2}\right]$ or [–90°, 90°]

It is important to determine if there is another angle in a different quadrant that also satisfies the problem. To do this, find the other quadrant(s) with the same sign for that trigonometric function and find the angle that has the same reference angle. Then check whether this angle is also a solution.
- In the first quadrant, all six trigonometric functions are positive (sin, cos, tan, csc, sec, cot).
- In the second quadrant, sin and csc are positive.
- In the third quadrant, tan and cot are positive.
- In the fourth quadrant, cos and sec are positive.

If you remember the phrase, "ALL Students Take Classes," you will be able to remember the sign of each trigonometric function in each quadrant. ALL represents all the signs in the first quadrant. The "S" in "Students" represents the sine function and its reciprocal in the second quadrant. The "T" in "Take" represents the tangent function and its reciprocal in the third quadrant. The "C" in "Classes" represents the cosine function and its reciprocal.

Trigonometric Identities

Sum and Difference
To find the sine, cosine, or tangent of the sum or difference of two angles, use one of the following formulas:
$$\sin(\alpha \pm \beta) = \sin \alpha \cos \beta \pm \cos \alpha \sin \beta$$
$$\cos(\alpha \pm \beta) = \cos \alpha \cos \beta \mp \sin \alpha \sin \beta$$
$$\tan(\alpha \pm \beta) = \frac{\tan \alpha \pm \tan \beta}{1 \mp \tan \alpha \tan \beta}$$
where α and β are two angles with known sine, cosine, or tangent values as needed.

Half angle
To find the sine or cosine of half of a known angle, use the following formulas:
$$\sin\frac{\theta}{2} = \pm\sqrt{\frac{1-\cos\theta}{2}}$$
$$\cos\frac{\theta}{2} = \pm\sqrt{\frac{1+\cos\theta}{2}}$$
where θ is an angle with a known exact cosine value.

To determine the sign of the answer, you must notice the quadrant the given angle is in and apply the correct sign for the trigonometric function you are using. If you need to find the exact sine or cosine of an angle that you do not know, such as sin 22.5°, you can rewrite the given angle as a half angle, such as $\sin\frac{45°}{2}$, and use the formula above.

To find the tangent or cotangent of half of a known angle, use the following formulas:
$$\tan\frac{\theta}{2} = \frac{\sin\theta}{1+\cos\theta}$$
$$\cot\frac{\theta}{2} = \frac{\sin\theta}{1-\cos\theta}$$
where θ is an angle with known exact sine and cosine values.

These formulas will work for finding the tangent or cotangent of half of any angle unless the cosine of θ happens to make the denominator of the identity equal to 0.

Double angles
In each case, use one of the Double Angle Formulas.
To find the sine or cosine of twice a known angle, use one of the following formulas:
$$\sin(2\theta) = 2\sin\theta\cos\theta$$
$$\cos(2\theta) = \cos^2\theta - \sin^2\theta \text{ or}$$
$$\cos(2\theta) = 2\cos^2\theta - 1 \text{ or}$$
$$\cos(2\theta) = 1 - 2\sin^2\theta$$

To find the tangent or cotangent of twice a known angle, use the formulas:
$$\tan(2\theta) = \frac{2\tan\theta}{1-\tan^2\theta}$$
$$\cot(2\theta) = \frac{\cot\theta - \tan\theta}{2}$$

In each case, θ is an angle with known exact sine, cosine, tangent, and cotangent values.

Products
To find the product of the sines and cosines of two different angles, use one of the following formulas:
$$\cos\alpha\cos\beta = \frac{1}{2}[\cos(\alpha+\beta) + \cos(\alpha-\beta)]$$
$$\sin\alpha\cos\beta = \frac{1}{2}[\sin(\alpha+\beta) + \sin(\alpha-\beta)]$$
$$\cos\alpha\sin\beta = \frac{1}{2}[\sin(\alpha+\beta) - \sin(\alpha-\beta)]$$
where α and β are two unique angles.

Complementary
The trigonometric cofunction identities use the trigonometric relationships of complementary angles (angles whose sum is 90°). These are:
$$\cos x = \sin(90° - x)$$
$$\csc x = \sec(90° - x)$$
$$\cot x = \tan(90° - x)$$

Pythagorean
The Pythagorean Theorem states that $a^2 + b^2 = c^2$ for all right triangles. The trigonometric identity that derives from this principle is stated in this way:
$$\sin^2\theta + \cos^2\theta = 1$$

Dividing each term by either $\sin^2\theta$ or $\cos^2\theta$ yields two other identities, respectively:
$$1 + \cot^2\theta = \csc^2\theta$$
$$\tan^2\theta + 1 = \sec^2\theta$$

Unit Circle

A unit circle is a circle with a radius of 1 that has its center at the origin. The equation of the unit circle is $x^2 + y^2 = 1$. Notice that this is an abbreviated version of the standard equation of a circle. Because the center is the point (0, 0), the values of h and k in the general equation are equal to zero and the equation simplifies to this form.

Standard Position is the position of an angle of measure θ whose vertex is at the origin, the initial side crosses the unit circle at the point (1, 0), and the terminal side crosses the unit circle at some other point (a, b). In the standard position, $\sin\theta = b$, $\cos\theta = a$, and $\tan\theta = \frac{b}{a}$.

Rectangular coordinates are those that lie on the square grids of the Cartesian plane. They should be quite familiar to you. The polar coordinate system is based on a circular graph, rather than the square grid of the Cartesian system. Points in the polar coordinate system are in the format (r, θ), where r is the distance from the origin (think radius of the circle) and θ is the smallest positive angle (moving counterclockwise around the circle) made with the positive horizontal axis.

To convert a point from rectangular (x, y) format to polar (r, θ) format, use the formula
$$(x, y) \text{ to } (r, \theta) \Rightarrow r = \sqrt{x^2 + y^2}; \theta = \arctan\frac{y}{x} \text{ when } x \neq 0$$

If x is positive, use the positive square root value for r. If x is negative, use the negative square root value for r.

If x = 0, use the following rules:
- If x = 0 and y = 0, then $\theta = 0$
- If x = 0 and y > 0, then $\theta = \frac{\pi}{2}$
- If x = 0 and y < 0, then $\theta = \frac{3\pi}{2}$

To convert a point from polar (r, θ) format to rectangular (x, y) format, use the formula
(r, θ) to $(x, y) \Rightarrow x = r\cos\theta; y = r\sin\theta$

Table of commonly encountered angles

$0° = 0$ radians, $30° = \frac{\pi}{6}$ radians, $45° = \frac{\pi}{4}$ radians, $60° = \frac{\pi}{3}$ radians, and $90° = \frac{\pi}{2}$ radians

$\sin 0° = 0$	$\cos 0° = 1$	$\tan 0° = 0$
$\sin 30° = \frac{1}{2}$	$\cos 30° = \frac{\sqrt{3}}{2}$	$\tan 30° = \frac{\sqrt{3}}{3}$
$\sin 45° = \frac{\sqrt{2}}{2}$	$\cos 45° = \frac{\sqrt{2}}{2}$	$\tan 45° = 1$
$\sin 60° = \frac{\sqrt{3}}{2}$	$\cos 60° = \frac{1}{2}$	$\tan 60° = \sqrt{3}$
$\sin 90° = 1$	$\cos 90° = 0$	$\tan 90° =$ undefined
$\csc 0° =$ undefined	$\sec 0° = 1$	$\cot 0° =$ undefined
$\csc 30° = 2$	$\sec 30° = \frac{2\sqrt{3}}{3}$	$\cot 30° = \sqrt{3}$
$\csc 45° = \sqrt{2}$	$\sec 45° = \sqrt{2}$	$\cot 45° = 1$
$\csc 60° = \frac{2\sqrt{3}}{3}$	$\sec 60° = 2$	$\cot 60° = \frac{\sqrt{3}}{3}$
$\csc 90° = 1$	$\sec 90° =$ undefined	$\cot 90° = 0$

The values in the upper half of this table are values you should have memorized or be able to find quickly.

The Reading Test

The 35 minute ACT Reading Test consists of four reading selections each followed by 10 questions. One of the four selections is drawn from the humanities, one from social studies, one from the natural sciences, and one from prose fiction.

Comprehension Skills

One of the most important skills in reading comprehension is the identification of **topics** and **main ideas.** There is a subtle difference between these two features. The topic is the subject of a text, or what the text is about. The main idea, on the other hand, is the most important point being made by the author. The topic is usually expressed in a few words at the most, while the main idea often needs a full sentence to be completely defined. As an example, a short passage might have the topic of penguins and the main idea *Penguins are different from other birds in many ways*. In most nonfiction writing, the topic and the main idea will be stated directly, often in a sentence at the very beginning or end of the text. When being tested on an understanding of the author's topic, the reader can quickly *skim* the passage for the general idea, stopping to read only the first sentence of each paragraph. A paragraph's first sentence is often (but not always) the main topic sentence, and it gives you a summary of the content of the paragraph. However, there are cases in which the reader must figure out an unstated topic or main idea. In these instances, the student must read every sentence of the text, and try to come up with an overarching idea that is supported by each of those sentences.

While the main idea is the overall premise of a story, **supporting details** provide evidence and backing for the main point. In order to show that a main idea is correct, or valid, the author needs to add details that prove their point. All texts contain details, but they are only classified as supporting details when they serve to reinforce some larger point. Supporting details are most commonly found in informative and persuasive texts. In some cases, they will be clearly indicated with words like *for example* or *for instance*, or they will be enumerated with words like *first*, *second*, and *last*. However, they may not be indicated with special words. As a reader, it is important to consider whether the author's supporting details really back up his or her main point. Supporting details can be factual and correct but still not relevant to the author's point. Conversely, supporting details can seem pertinent but be ineffective because they are based on opinion or assertions that cannot be proven.

An example of a main idea is: "Giraffes live in the Serengeti of Africa." A supporting detail about giraffes could be: "A giraffe uses its long neck to reach twigs and leaves on trees." The main idea gives the general idea that the text is about giraffes. The supporting detail gives a specific fact about how the giraffes eat.

As opposed to a main idea, themes are seldom expressed directly in a text, so they can be difficult to identify. A **theme** is an issue, an idea, or a question raised by the text. For instance, a theme of William Shakespeare's *Hamlet* is indecision, as the title character explores his own psyche and the results of his failure to make bold choices. A great work of literature may have many themes, and the reader is justified in identifying any for which he or she can find support. One common characteristic of themes is that they raise more questions than they answer. In a good piece of fiction, the author is not always trying to convince the reader, but is instead trying to elevate the reader's perspective and encourage him to consider the themes more deeply. When reading, one can identify themes by constantly asking what general issues the text is addressing. A good way to evaluate an author's approach to a theme is to begin reading with a question in mind (for example, how does this text approach the theme of love?) and then look for evidence in the text that addresses that question.

Purposes for Writing

In order to be an effective reader, one must pay attention to the author's **position** and purpose. Even those texts that seem objective and impartial, like textbooks, have some sort of position and bias. Readers need to take these positions into account when considering the author's message. When an author uses emotional language or clearly favors one side of an argument, his position is clear. However, the author's position may be evident not only in what he writes, but in what he doesn't write. For this reason, it is sometimes necessary to review some other texts on the same topic in order to develop a view of the author's position. If this is not possible, then it may be useful to acquire a little background personal information about the author. When the only source of information is the text, however, the reader should look for language and argumentation that seems to indicate a particular stance on the subject.

Identifying the **purpose** of an author is usually easier than identifying her position. In most cases, the author has no interest in hiding his or her purpose. A text that is meant to entertain, for instance, should be obviously written to please the reader. Most narratives, or stories, are written to entertain, though they may also inform or persuade. Informative texts are easy to identify as well. The most difficult purpose of a text to identify is persuasion, because the author has an interest in making this purpose hard to detect. When a person knows that the author is trying to convince him, he is automatically more wary and skeptical of the argument. For this reason persuasive texts often try to establish an entertaining tone, hoping to amuse the reader into agreement, or an informative tone, hoping to create an appearance of authority and objectivity.

An author's purpose is often evident in the organization of the text. For instance, if the text has headings and subheadings, if key terms are in bold, and if the author makes his main idea clear from the beginning, then the likely purpose of the text is to inform. If the author begins by making a claim and then makes various arguments to support that claim, the purpose is probably to persuade. If the author is telling a story, or is more interested in holding the attention of the reader than in making a particular point or delivering information, then his purpose is most likely to entertain. As a reader, it is best to judge an author on how well he accomplishes his purpose. In other words, it is not entirely fair to complain that a textbook is boring: if the text is clear and easy to understand, then the author has done his job. Similarly, a storyteller should not be judged too harshly for getting some facts wrong, so long as he is able to give pleasure to the reader.

The author's purpose for writing will affect his writing style and the response of the reader. In a **persuasive essay**, the author is attempting to change the reader's mind or convince him of something he did not believe previously. There are several identifying characteristics of persuasive writing. One is opinion presented as fact. When an author attempts to persuade the reader, he often presents his or her opinions as if they were fact. A reader must be on guard for statements that sound factual but which cannot be subjected to research, observation, or experiment. Another characteristic of persuasive writing is emotional language. An author will often try to play on the reader's emotion by appealing to his sympathy or sense of morality. When an author uses colorful or evocative language with the intent of arousing the reader's passions, it is likely that he is attempting to persuade. Finally, in many cases a persuasive text will give an unfair explanation of opposing positions, if these positions are mentioned at all.

An **informative text** is written to educate and enlighten the reader. Informative texts are almost always nonfiction, and are rarely structured as a story. The intention of an informative text is to deliver information in the most comprehensible way possible, so the structure of the text is likely to be very clear. In an informative text, the thesis statement is often in the first sentence. The author may use some colorful language, but is likely to put more emphasis on clarity and precision. Informative essays do not typically appeal to the emotions. They often contain facts and figures, and rarely include the opinion of the author. Sometimes a persuasive essay can resemble an informative essay, especially if the author maintains an even tone and presents his or her views as if they were established fact.

The success or failure of an author's intent to **entertain** is determined by those who read the author's work. Entertaining texts may be either fiction or nonfiction, and they may describe real or imagined people, places, and events. Entertaining texts are often narratives, or stories. A text that is written to entertain is likely to contain colorful language that engages the imagination and the emotions. Such writing often features a great deal of figurative language, which typically enlivens its subject matter with images and analogies. Though an entertaining text is not usually written to persuade or inform, it may accomplish both of these tasks. An entertaining text may appeal to the reader's emotions and cause him or her to think differently about a particular subject. In any case, entertaining texts tend to showcase the personality of the author more so than do other types of writing.

When an author intends to **express feelings,** she may use colorful and evocative language. An author may write emotionally for any number of reasons. Sometimes, the author will do so because she is describing a personal situation of great pain or happiness. Sometimes an author is attempting to persuade the reader, and so will use emotion to stir up the passions. It can be easy to identify this kind of expression when the writer uses phrases like *I felt* and *I sense*. However, sometimes the author will simply describe feelings without introducing them. As a reader, it is important to recognize when an author is expressing emotion, and not to become overwhelmed by sympathy or passion. A reader should maintain some detachment so that he or she can still evaluate the strength of the author's argument or the quality of the writing.

In a sense, almost all writing is descriptive, insofar as it seeks to describe events, ideas, or people to the reader. Some texts, however, are primarily concerned with **description**. A descriptive text focuses on a particular subject, and attempts to depict it in a way that will be clear to the reader. Descriptive texts contain many adjectives and adverbs, words that give shades of meaning and create a more detailed mental picture for the reader. A descriptive text fails when it is unclear or vague to the reader. On the other hand, however, a descriptive text that compiles too much detail can be boring and overwhelming to the reader. A descriptive text will certainly be informative, and it may be persuasive and entertaining as well. Descriptive writing is a challenge for the author, but when it is done well, it can be fun to read.

Writing Devices

Authors will use different stylistic and writing devices to make their meaning more clearly understood. One of those devices is comparison and contrast. When an author describes the ways in which two things are alike, he or she is **comparing** them. When the author describes the ways in which two things are different, he or she is **contrasting** them. The "compare and contrast" essay is one of the most common forms in nonfiction. It is often signaled with certain words: a comparison may be indicated with such words as *both*, *same*, *like*, *too*, and *as well*; while a contrast may be indicated by words like *but*, *however*, *on the other hand*, *instead*, and *yet*. Of course, comparisons and contrasts may be implicit without using any such signaling language. A single sentence may both compare and contrast. Consider the sentence *Brian and Sheila love ice cream, but Brian prefers vanilla and Sheila prefers strawberry*. In one sentence, the author has described both a similarity (love of ice cream) and a difference (favorite flavor).

One of the most common text structures is **cause and effect**. A cause is an act or event that makes something happen, and an effect is the thing that happens as a result of that cause. A cause-and-effect relationship is not always explicit, but there are some words in English that signal causality, such as *since*, *because*, and *as a result*. As an example, consider the sentence *Because the sky was clear, Ron did not bring an umbrella*. The cause is the clear sky, and the effect is that Ron did not bring an umbrella. However, sometimes the cause-and-effect relationship will not be clearly noted. For instance, the sentence *He was late and missed the meeting* does not contain any signaling words, but it still contains a cause (he was late) and an effect (he missed the meeting). It is possible for a single cause to have multiple effects, or for a single effect to have multiple causes. Also, an effect can in turn be the cause of another effect, in what is known as a cause-and-effect chain.

Authors often use analogies to add meaning to the text. An **analogy** is a comparison of two things. The words in the analogy are connected by a certain, often undetermined relationship. Look at this analogy: moo is to cow as quack is to duck. This analogy compares the sound that a cow makes with the sound that a duck makes. Even if the word 'quack' was not given, one could figure out it is the correct word to complete the analogy based on the relationship between the words 'moo' and 'cow'. Some common relationships for analogies include synonyms, antonyms, part to whole, definition, and actor to action.

Another element that impacts a text is the author's point of view. The **point of view** of a text is the perspective from which it is told. The author will always have a point of view about a story before he draws up a plot line. The author will know what events they want to take place, how they want the characters to interact, and how the story will resolve. An author will also have an opinion on the topic, or series of events, which is presented in the story, based on their own prior experience and beliefs.

The two main points of view that authors use are first person and third person. If the narrator of the story is also the main character, or *protagonist*, the text is written in first-person point of view. In first person, the author writes with the word *I*. Third-person point of view is probably the most common point of view that authors use. Using third person, authors refer to each character using the words *he* or *she*. In third-person omniscient, the narrator is not a character in the story and tells the story of all of the characters at the same time.

A good writer will use **transitional words** and phrases to guide the reader through the text. You are no doubt familiar with the common transitions, though you may never have considered how they operate. Some transitional phrases (*after, before, during, in the middle of*) give information about time. Some indicate that an example is about to be given (*for example, in fact, for instance*). Writers use them to compare (*also, likewise*) and contrast (*however, but, yet*). Transitional words and phrases can suggest addition (*and, also, furthermore, moreover*) and logical relationships (*if, then, therefore, as a result, since*). Finally, transitional words and phrases can demarcate the steps in a process (*first, second, last*). You should incorporate transitional words and phrases where they will orient your reader and illuminate the structure of your composition.

Types of Passages

A **narrative** passage is a story. Narratives can be fiction or nonfiction. However, there are a few elements that a text must have in order to be classified as a narrative. To begin with, the text must have a plot. That is, it must describe a series of events. If it is a good narrative, these events will be interesting and emotionally engaging to the reader. A narrative also has characters. These could be people, animals, or even inanimate objects, so long as they participate in the plot. A narrative passage often contains figurative language, which is meant to stimulate the imagination of the reader by making comparisons and observations. A metaphor, which is a description of one thing in terms of another, is a common piece of figurative language. *The moon was a frosty snowball* is an example of a metaphor: it is obviously untrue in the literal sense, but it suggests a certain mood for the reader. Narratives often proceed in a clear sequence, but they do not need to do so.

An **expository** passage aims to inform and enlighten the reader. It is nonfiction and usually centers around a simple, easily defined topic. Since the goal of exposition is to teach, such a passage should be as clear as possible. It is common for an expository passage to contain helpful organizing words, like *first, next, for example*, and *therefore*. These words keep the reader oriented in the text. Although expository passages do not need to feature colorful language and artful writing, they are often more effective when they do. For a reader, the challenge of expository passages is to maintain steady attention. Expository passages are not always about subjects in which a reader will naturally be interested, and the writer is often more concerned with clarity and comprehensibility than with engaging the reader. For this reason, many expository passages are dull. Making notes is a good way to maintain focus when reading an expository passage.

A **technical** passage is written to describe a complex object or process. Technical writing is common in medical and technological fields, in which complicated mathematical, scientific, and engineering ideas need to be explained simply and clearly. To ease comprehension, a technical passage usually proceeds in a very logical order. Technical passages often have clear headings and subheadings, which are used to keep the reader oriented in the text. It is also common for these passages to break sections up with numbers or letters. Many technical passages look more like an outline than a piece of prose. The amount of jargon or difficult vocabulary will vary in a technical passage depending on the intended audience. As much as possible, technical passages try to avoid language that the reader will have to research in order to understand the message. Of course, it is not always possible to avoid jargon.

A **persuasive** passage is meant to change the reader's mind or lead her into agreement with the author. The persuasive intent may be obvious, or it may be quite difficult to discern. In some cases, a persuasive passage will be indistinguishable from an informative passage: it will make an assertion and offer supporting details. However, a persuasive passage is more likely to make claims based on opinion and to appeal to the reader's emotions. Persuasive passages may not describe alternate positions and, when they do, they often display significant bias. It may be clear that a persuasive passage is giving the author's viewpoint, or the passage may adopt a seemingly objective tone. A persuasive passage is successful if it can make a convincing argument and win the trust of the reader.

A persuasive essay will likely focus on one central argument, but it may make many smaller claims along the way. These are subordinate arguments with which the reader must agree if he or she is going to agree with the central argument. The central argument will only be as strong as the subordinate claims. These claims should be rooted in fact and observation, rather than subjective judgment. The best persuasive essays provide enough supporting detail to justify claims without overwhelming the reader. Remember that a fact must be susceptible to independent verification: that is, it must be something the reader could confirm. Also, statistics are only effective when they take into account possible objections. For instance, a statistic on the number of foreclosed houses would only be useful if it was taken over a defined interval and in a defined area. Most readers are wary of statistics, because they are so often misleading. If possible, a persuasive essay should always include references so that the reader can obtain more information. Of course, this means that the writer's accuracy and fairness may be judged by the inquiring reader.

Opinions are formed by emotion as well as reason, and persuasive writers often appeal to the feelings of the reader. Although readers should always be skeptical of this technique, it is often used in a proper and ethical manner. For instance, there are many subjects that have an obvious emotional component, and therefore cannot be completely treated without an appeal to the emotions. Consider an article on drunk driving: it makes sense to include some specific examples that will alarm or sadden the reader. After all, drunk driving often has serious and tragic consequences. Emotional appeals are not appropriate, however, when they attempt to mislead the reader. For instance, in political advertisements it is common to emphasize the patriotism of the preferred candidate, because this will encourage the audience to link their own positive feelings about the country with their opinion of the candidate. However, these ads often imply that the other candidate is unpatriotic, which in most cases is far from the truth. Another common and improper emotional appeal is the use of loaded language, as for instance referring to an avidly religious person as a "fanatic" or a passionate environmentalist as a "tree hugger." These terms introduce an emotional component that detracts from the argument.

History and Culture

Historical context has a profound influence on literature: the events, knowledge base, and assumptions of an author's time color every aspect of his or her work. Sometimes, authors hold opinions and use language that would be considered inappropriate or immoral in a modern setting, but that was acceptable in the author's time. As a reader, one should consider how the historical context influenced a work and also how today's opinions and ideas shape the way modern readers read the works of the past. For instance, in most societies of the past, women were treated as second-class citizens. An author who wrote in 18th-century England might sound sexist to modern readers, even if that author was relatively feminist in his time. Readers should not have to excuse the faulty assumptions and prejudices of the past, but they should appreciate that a person's thoughts and words are, in part, a result of the time and culture in which they live or lived, and it is perhaps unfair to expect writers to avoid all of the errors of their times.

Even a brief study of world literature suggests that writers from vastly different cultures address similar themes. For instance, works like the *Odyssey* and *Hamlet* both tackle the individual's battle for self-control and independence. In every culture, authors address themes of personal growth and the struggle for maturity. Another universal theme is the conflict between the individual and society. In works as culturally disparate as *Native Son*, the *Aeneid*, and *1984*, authors dramatize how people struggle to maintain their personalities and dignity in large, sometimes oppressive groups. Finally, many cultures have versions of the hero's (or heroine's) journey, in which an adventurous person must overcome many obstacles in order to gain greater knowledge, power, and perspective. Some famous works that treat this theme are the *Epic of Gilgamesh*, Dante's *Divine Comedy*, and *Don Quixote*.

Authors from different genres (for instance poetry, drama, novel, short story) and cultures may address similar themes, but they often do so quite differently. For instance, poets are likely to address subject matter obliquely, through the use of images and allusions. In a play, on the other hand, the author is more likely to dramatize themes by using characters to express opposing viewpoints. This disparity is known as a dialectical approach. In a novel, the author does not need to express themes directly; rather, they can be illustrated through events and actions. In some regional literatures, like those of Greece or England, authors use more irony: their works have characters that express views and make decisions that are clearly disapproved of by the author. In Latin America, there is a great tradition of using supernatural events to illustrate themes about real life. In China and Japan, authors frequently use well-established regional forms (haiku, for instance) to organize their treatment of universal themes.

Responding to Literature

When reading good literature, the reader is moved to engage actively in the text. One part of being an active reader involves making predictions. A **prediction** is a guess about what will happen next. Readers are constantly making predictions based on what they have read and what they already know. Consider the following sentence: *Staring at the computer screen in shock, Kim blindly reached over for the brimming glass of water on the shelf to her side.* The sentence suggests that Kim is agitated and that she is not looking at the glass she is going to pick up, so a reader might predict that she is going to knock the glass over. Of course, not every prediction will be accurate: perhaps Kim will pick the glass up cleanly. Nevertheless, the author has certainly created the expectation that the water might be spilled. Predictions are always subject to revision as the reader acquires more information.

Test-taking tip: To respond to questions requiring future predictions, the student's answers should be based on evidence of past or present behavior.

Readers are often required to understand text that claims and suggests ideas without stating them directly. An **inference** is a piece of information that is implied but not written outright by the author. For instance, consider the following sentence: *Mark made more money that week than he* *had in the previous year*. From this sentence, the reader can infer that Mark either has not made much money in the previous year or made a great deal of money that week. Often, a reader can use information he or she already knows to make inferences. Take as an example the sentence *When his coffee arrived, he looked around the table for the silver cup.* Many people know that cream is typically served in a silver cup, so using their own base of knowledge they can infer that the subject of this sentence takes his coffee with cream. Making inferences requires concentration, attention, and practice.

Test-taking tip: While being tested on his ability to make correct inferences, the student must look for contextual clues. An answer can be *true* but not *correct*. The contextual clues will help you find the answer that is the best answer out of the given choices. Understand the context in which a phrase is stated. When asked for the implied meaning of a statement made in the passage, the student should immediately locate the statement and read the context in which it was made. Also, look for an answer choice that has a similar phrase to the statement in question.

A reader must be able to identify a text's **sequence**, or the order in which things happen. Often, and especially when the sequence is very important to the author, it is indicated with signal words like *first, then, next,* and *last*. However, sometimes a sequence is merely implied and must be noted by the reader. Consider the sentence *He walked in the front door and switched on the hall lamp.* Clearly, the man did not turn the lamp on before he walked in the door, so the implied sequence is that he first walked in the door and then turned on the lamp. Texts do not always proceed in an orderly sequence from first to last: sometimes, they begin at the end and then start over at the beginning. As a reader, it can be useful to make brief notes to clarify the sequence.

In addition to inferring and predicting things about the text, the reader must often **draw conclusions** about the information he has read. When asked for a *conclusion* that may be drawn, look for critical "hedge" phrases, such as *likely, may, can, will often,* among many others.

When you are being tested on this knowledge, remember that question writers insert these hedge phrases to cover every possibility. Often an answer will be wrong simply because it leaves no room for exception. Extreme positive or negative answers (such as always, never, etc.) are usually not correct. The reader should not use any outside knowledge that is not gathered from the reading passage to answer the related questions. Correct answers can be derived straight from the reading passage.

Literary Genres

Literary genres refer to the basic generic types of poetry, drama, fiction, and nonfiction. Literary genre is a method of classifying and analyzing literature. There are numerous subdivisions within genre, including such categories as novels, novellas, and short stories in fiction. Drama may also be subdivided into comedy, tragedy, and many other categories. Poetry and nonfiction have their own distinct divisions.

Genres often overlap, and the distinctions among them are blurred, such as that between the nonfiction novel and docudrama, as well as many others. However, the use of genres is helpful to the reader as a set of understandings that guide our responses to a work. The generic norm sets expectations and forms the framework within which we read and evaluate a work. This framework will guide both our understanding and interpretation of the work. It is a useful tool for both literary criticism and analysis.

Fiction is a general term for any form of literary narrative that is invented or imagined rather than being factual. For those individuals who equate fact with truth, the imagined or invented character of fiction tends to render it relatively unimportant or trivial among the genres. Defenders of fiction are quick to point out that the fictional mode is an essential part of being. The ability to imagine or discuss what-if plots, characters, and events is clearly part of the human experience.

Prose is derived from the Latin and means "straightforward discourse." Prose fiction, although having many categories, may be divided into three main groups:
- **Short stories**: a fictional narrative, the length of which varies, usually under 20,000 words. Short stories usually have only a few characters and generally describe one major event or insight. The short story began in magazines in the late 1800s and has flourished ever since.
- **Novels**: a longer work of fiction, often containing a large cast of characters and extensive plotting. The emphasis may be on an event, action, social problems, or any experience. There is now a genre of nonfiction novels pioneered by Truman Capote's *In Cold Blood* in the 1960s. Novels may also be written in verse.
- **Novellas**: a work of narrative fiction longer than a short story but shorter than a novel. Novellas may also be called short novels or novelettes. They originated from the German tradition and have become common forms in all of the world's literature.

Many elements influence a work of prose fiction. Some important ones are:
- Speech and dialogue: Characters may speak for themselves or through the narrator. Dialogue may be realistic or fantastic, depending on the author's aim.
- Thoughts and mental processes: There may be internal dialogue used as a device for plot development or character understanding.
- Dramatic involvement: Some narrators encourage readers to become involved in the events of the story, whereas others attempt to distance readers through literary devices.
- Action: This is any information that advances the plot or involves new interactions between the characters.
- Duration: The time frame of the work may be long or short, and the relationship between described time and narrative time may vary.
- Setting and description: Is the setting critical to the plot or characters? How are the action scenes described?
- Themes: This is any point of view or topic given sustained attention.
- Symbolism: Authors often veil meanings through imagery and other literary constructions.

Fiction is much wider than simply prose fiction. Songs, ballads, epics, and narrative poems are examples of non-prose fiction. A full definition of fiction must include not only the work itself but also the framework in which it is read. Literary fiction can also be defined as not true rather than nonexistent, as many works of historical fiction refer to real people, places, and events that are treated imaginatively as if they were true. These imaginary elements enrich and broaden literary expression.

When analyzing fiction, it is important for the reader to look carefully at the work being studied. The plot or action of a narrative can become so entertaining that the language of the work is ignored. The language of fiction should not simply be a way to relate a plot—it should also yield many insights to the judicious reader. Some prose fiction is based on the reader's engagement with the language rather than the story. A studious reader will analyze the mode of expression as well as the narrative. Part of the reward of reading in this manner is to discover how the author uses different language to describe familiar objects, events, or emotions. Some works focus the reader on an author's unorthodox use of language, whereas others may emphasize characters or storylines. What happens in a story is not always the critical element in the work. This type of reading may be difficult at first but yields great rewards.

The **narrator** is a central part of any work of fiction, and can give insight about the purpose of the work and its main themes and ideas. The following are important questions to address to better understand the voice and role of the narrator and incorporate that voice into an overall understanding of the novel:

- Who is the narrator of the novel? What is the narrator's perspective, first person or third person? What is the role of the narrator in the plot? Are there changes in narrators or the perspective of narrators?
- Does the narrator explain things in the novel, or does meaning emerge from the plot and events? The personality of the narrator is important. She may have a vested interest in a character or event described. Some narratives follow the time sequence of the plot, whereas others do not. A narrator may express approval or disapproval about a character or events in the work.
- Tone is an important aspect of the narration. Who is actually being addressed by the narrator? Is the tone familiar or formal, intimate or impersonal? Does the vocabulary suggest clues about the narrator?

A **character** is a person intimately involved with the plot and development of the novel. Development of the novel's characters not only moves the story along but will also tell the reader a lot about the novel itself. There is usually a physical description of the character, but this is often omitted in modern and postmodern novels. These works may focus on the psychological state or motivation of the character. The choice of a character's name may give valuable clues to his role in the work.

Characters are said to be flat or round. Flat characters tend to be minor figures in the story, changing little or not at all. Round characters (those understood from a well-rounded view) are more central to the story and tend to change as the plot unfolds. Stock characters are similar to flat characters, filling out the story without influencing it.

Modern literature has been greatly affected by Freudian psychology, giving rise to such devices as the interior monologue and magical realism as methods of understanding characters in a work. These give the reader a more complex understanding of the inner lives of the characters and enrich the understanding of relationships between characters.

Another important genre is that of **drama**: a play written to be spoken aloud. The drama is in many ways inseparable from performance. Reading drama ideally involves using imagination to visualize and re-create the play with characters and settings. The reader stages the play in his imagination, watching characters interact and developments unfold. Sometimes this involves simulating a theatrical presentation; other times it involves imagining the events. In either case, the reader is imagining the unwritten to re-create the dramatic experience. Novels present some of the same problems, but a narrator will provide much more information about the setting, characters, inner dialogues, and many other supporting details. In drama, much of this is missing, and we are required to use our powers of projection and imagination to taste the full flavor of the dramatic work. There are many empty spaces in dramatic texts that must be filled by the reader to fully appreciate the work.

When reading drama in this way, there are some advantages over watching the play performed (though there is much criticism in this regard):

- Freedom of point of view and perspective: Text is free of interpretations of actors, directors, producers, and technical staging.
- Additional information: The text of a drama may be accompanied by notes or prefaces placing the work in a social or historical context. Stage directions may also provide relevant information about the author's purpose. None of this is typically available at live or filmed performances.
- Study and understanding: Difficult or obscure passages may be studied at leisure and supplemented by explanatory works. This is particularly true of older plays with unfamiliar language, which cannot be fully understood without an opportunity to study the material.

Critical elements of drama, especially when it is being read aloud or performed, include dialect, speech, and dialogue. Analysis of speech and dialogue is important in the critical study of drama. Some playwrights use speech to develop their characters. Speeches may be long or short, and written in as normal prose or blank verse. Some characters have a unique way of speaking which illuminates aspects of the drama. Emphasis and tone are both important, as well. Does the author make clear the tone in which lines are to be spoken, or is this open to interpretation? Sometimes there are various possibilities in tone with regard to delivering lines.

Dialect is any distinct variety of a language, especially one spoken in a region or part of a country. The criterion for distinguishing dialects from languages is that of mutual understanding. For example, people who speak Dutch cannot understand English unless they have learned it. But a speaker from Amsterdam can understand one from Antwerp; therefore, they speak different dialects of the same language. This is, however, a matter of degree; there are languages in which different dialects are unintelligible.

Dialect mixtures are the presence in one form of speech with elements from different neighboring dialects. The study of speech differences from one geographical area to another is called dialect geography. A dialect atlas is a map showing distribution of dialects in a given area. A dialect continuum shows a progressive shift in dialects across a territory, such that adjacent dialects are understandable, but those at the extremes are not.

Dramatic dialogue can be difficult to interpret and changes depending upon the tone used and which words are emphasized. Where the stresses, or meters, of dramatic dialogue fall can determine meaning. Variations in emphasis are only one factor in the manipulability of dramatic speech. Tone is of equal or greater importance and expresses a range of possible emotions and feelings that cannot be readily discerned from the script of a play. The reader must add tone to the words to understand the full meaning of a passage. Recognizing tone is a cumulative process as the reader begins to understand the characters and situations in the play. Other elements that influence the interpretation of dialogue include the setting, possible reactions of the characters to the speech, and possible gestures or facial expressions of the actor. There are no firm rules to guide the interpretation of dramatic speech. An open and flexible attitude is essential in interpreting dramatic dialogue.

Action is a crucial element in the production of a dramatic work. Many dramas contain little dialogue and much action. In these cases, it is essential for the reader to carefully study stage directions and visualize the action on the stage. Benefits of understanding stage directions include knowing which characters are on the stage at all times, who is speaking to whom, and following these patterns through changes of scene.

Stage directions also provide additional information, some of which is not available to a live audience. The nature of the physical space where the action occurs is vital, and stage directions help with this. The historical context of the period is important in understanding what the playwright was working with in terms of theaters and physical space. The type of staging possible for the author is a good guide to the spatial elements of a production.

Asides and soliloquies are devices that authors use in plot and character development. **Asides** indicate that not all characters are privy to the lines. This may be a method of advancing or explaining the plot in a subtle manner. **Soliloquies** are opportunities for character development, plot enhancement, and to give insight to characters motives, feelings, and emotions. Careful study of these elements provides a reader with an abundance of clues to the major themes and plot of the work.

Art, music, and literature all interact in ways that contain many opportunities for the enrichment of all of the arts. Students could apply their knowledge of art and music by creating illustrations for a work or creating a musical score for a text. Students could discuss the meanings of texts and decide on their illustrations, or a score could amplify the meaning of the text.

Understanding the art and music of a period can make the experience of literature a richer, more rewarding experience. Students should be encouraged to use the knowledge of art and music to illuminate the text. Examining examples of dress, architecture, music, and dance of a period may be helpful in a fuller engagement of the text. Much of period literature lends itself to the analysis of the prevailing taste in art and music of an era, which helps place the literary work in a more meaningful context.

Testing Tips

Skimming

Your first task when you begin reading is to answer the question "What is the topic of the selection?" This can best be answered by quickly skimming the passage for the general idea, stopping to read only the first sentence of each paragraph. A paragraph's first is usually the main topic sentence, and it gives you a summary of the content of the paragraph.

Once you've skimmed the passage, stopping to read only the first sentences, you will have a general idea about what it is about, as well as what is the expected topic in each paragraph.

Each question will contain clues as to where to find the answer in the passage. Do not just randomly search through the passage for the correct answer to each question. Search scientifically. Find key word(s) or ideas in the question that are going to either contain or be near the correct answer. These are typically nouns, verbs, numbers, or phrases in the question that will probably be duplicated in the passage. Once you have identified those key word(s) or idea, skim the passage quickly to find where those key word(s) or idea appears. The correct answer choice will be nearby.

Example: What caused Martin to suddenly return to Paris?

The key word is Paris. Skim the passage quickly to find where this word appears. The answer will be close by that word.

However, sometimes key words in the question are not repeated in the passage. In those cases, search for the general idea of the question.

Example: Which of the following was the psychological impact of the author's childhood upon the remainder of his life?

Key words are "childhood" or "psychology". While searching for those words, be alert for other words or phrases that have similar meaning, such as "emotional effect" or "mentally" which could be used in the passage, rather than the exact word "psychology".

Numbers or years can be particularly good keywords to skim for, as they stand out from the rest of the text.

Example: Which of the following best describes the influence of Monet's work in the 20th century?

20th contains numbers and will easily stand out from the rest of the text. Use *20th* as the keyword to skim for in the passage.

Other good key word(s) may be in quotation marks. These identify a word or phrase that is copied directly from the passage. In those cases, the word(s) in quotation marks are exactly duplicated in the passage.

Example: In her college years, what was meant by Margaret's "drive for excellence"?

"Drive for excellence" is a direct quote from the passage and should be easy to find.

Once you've quickly found the correct section of the passage to find the answer, focus upon the answer choices. Sometimes a choice will repeat word for word a portion of the passage near the answer. However, beware of such duplication – it may be a trap! More than likely, the correct choice will paraphrase or summarize the related portion of the passage, rather than being exactly the same wording.

For the answers that you think are correct, read them carefully and make sure that they answer the question. An answer can be factually correct, but it MUST answer the question asked. Additionally, two answers can both be seemingly correct, so be sure to read all of the answer choices, and make sure that you get the one that BEST answers the question.

Some questions will not have a key word.

Example: Which of the following would the author of this passage likely agree with?

In these cases, look for key words in the answer choices. Then skim the passage to find where the answer choice occurs. By skimming to find where to look, you can minimize the time required.

Sometimes it may be difficult to identify a good key word in the question to skim for in the passage. In those cases, look for a key word in one of the answer choices to skim for. Often the answer choices can all be found in the same paragraph, which can quickly narrow your search.

Paragraph Focus

Focus upon the first sentence of each paragraph, which is the most important. The main topic of the paragraph is usually there.

Once you've read the first sentence in the paragraph, you have a general idea about what each paragraph will be about. As you read the questions, try to determine which paragraph will have the answer. Paragraphs have a concise topic. The answer should either obviously be there or obviously not. It will save time if you can jump straight to the paragraph, so try to remember what you learned from the first sentences.

Example: The first paragraph is about poets; the second is about poetry. If a question asks about poetry, where will the answer be? *The second paragraph.*

The main idea of a passage is typically spread across all or most of its paragraphs. Whereas the main idea of a paragraph may be completely different than the main idea of the very next paragraph, a main idea for a passage affects all of the paragraphs in one form or another.
Example: What is the main idea of the passage?

For each answer choice, try to see how many paragraphs are related. It can help to count how many sentences are affected by each choice, but it is best to see how many paragraphs are affected by the choice. Typically the answer choices will include incorrect choices that are main ideas of individual paragraphs, but not the entire passage. That is why it is crucial to choose ideas that are supported by the most paragraphs possible.

Eliminate Choices

Some choices can quickly be eliminated. "Andy Warhol lived there." Is Andy Warhol even mentioned in the article? If not, quickly eliminate it.

When trying to answer a question such as "the passage indicates all of the following EXCEPT" quickly skim the paragraph searching for references to each choice. If the reference exists, scratch it off as a choice. Similar choices may be crossed off simultaneously if they are close enough.

In choices that ask you to choose "which answer choice does NOT describe?" or "all of the following answer choices are identifiable characteristics, EXCEPT which?" look for answers that are similarly worded. Since only one answer can be correct, if there are two answers that appear to mean the same thing, they must BOTH be incorrect, and can be eliminated.

Example Answer Choices:
A. changing values and attitudes
B. a large population of mobile or uprooted people

These answer choices are similar; they both describe a fluid culture. Because of their similarity, they can be linked together. Since the answer can have only one choice, they can also be eliminated together.

When presented with a question that offers two choices, or neither choice, or both choice, it is rarely both choices.

Example: When an atom emits a beta particle, the mass of the atom will:
A. increase
B. decrease.
C. stay the same.
D. either increase or decrease depending on conditions.

Answer D will rarely be correct, the answers are usually more concrete.

Contextual Clues

Look for contextual clues. An answer can be right but not correct. The contextual clues will help you find the answer that is most right and is correct. Understand the context in which a phrase is stated.

When asked for the implied meaning of a statement made in the passage, immediately go find the statement and read the context it was made in. Also, look for an answer choice that has a similar phrase to the statement in question.

Example: In the passage, what is implied by the phrase "Churches have become more or less part of the furniture"?

Find an answer choice that is similar or describes the phrase "part of the furniture" as that is the key phrase in the question. "Part of the furniture" is a saying that means something is fixed, immovable, or set in their ways. Those are all similar ways of saying "part of the furniture." As such, the correct answer choice will probably include a similar rewording of the expression.

Example: Why was John described as "morally desperate"?

The answer will probably have some sort of definition of morals in it. "Morals" refers to a code of right and wrong behavior, so the correct answer choice will likely have words that mean something like that.

Fact/Opinion

When asked about which statement is a fact or opinion, remember that answer choices that are facts will typically have no ambiguous words. For example, how long is a long time? What defines an ordinary person? These ambiguous words of "long" and "ordinary" should not be in a factual statement. However, if all of the choices have ambiguous words, go to the context of the passage. Often a factual statement may be set out as a research finding.

Example: "The scientist found that the eye reacts quickly to change in light."

Opinions may be set out in the context of words like thought, believed, understood, or wished.

Example: "He thought the Yankees should win the World Series."

Time Management

In technical passages, do not get lost on the technical terms. Skip them and move on. You want a general understanding of what is going on, not a mastery of the passage.

When you encounter material in the selection that seems difficult to understand, bracket it. It often may not be necessary and can be skipped. Only spend time trying to understand it if it is going to be relevant for a question. Understand difficult phrases only as a last resort.

If low on time, save sequence questions that ask you to sequence four choices (I, II, III, IV) for last. They consume a lot of time. When you do work on them, first find the four sequences in the passages, and mark them I, II, III, and IV respectively. Look for transitional word cues in the sentences such as: first, initially, to start, early on, finally, in conclusion, in the end, or last. These transition words can help position the choices. Also, focus on eliminating the wrong choices. If you know that a certain sequence must be first or last, then you can eliminate the choices that do not have that as an option.

Pace yourself. 9 minutes per passage, which is nearly a minute per question.
Do easy passages and questions first. The easier passages should be first.

Answer general questions before detail questions. A reader with a good understanding of the whole passage can often answer general questions without rereading a word. Get the easier questions out of the way before tackling the more time consuming ones.

Identify each question by type. Usually the wording of a question will tell you whether you can find the answer by referring directly to the passage or by using your reasoning powers. You alone know which question types you customarily handle with ease and which give you trouble and will require more time. Save the difficult questions for last.

Warnings

When asked for a conclusion that may be drawn, look for critical "hedge" phrases, such as likely, may, can, will often, sometimes, etc, often, almost, mostly, usually, generally, rarely, sometimes. Question writers insert these hedge phrases, to cover every possibility. Often an answer will be wrong simply because it leaves no room for exception.

Example: Animals live longer in cold places than animals in warm places.

This answer choice is wrong, because there are exceptions in which certain warm climate animals live longer. This answer choice leaves no possibility of exception. It states that every animal species in cold places live longer than animal species in warm places. Correct answer choices will typically have a key hedge word to leave room for exceptions.

Example: In severe cold, a polar bear cub is likely to survive longer than an adult polar bear.

This answer choice is correct, because not only does the passage imply that younger animals survive better in the cold, it also allows for exceptions to exist. The use of the word "likely" leaves room for cases in which a polar bear cub might not survive longer than the adult polar bear.

When asked how a word is used in the passage, don't use your existing knowledge of the word. The question is being asked precisely because there is some strange or unusual usage of the word in the passage. Go to the passage and use contextual clues to determine the answer. Don't simply use the popular definition you already know.

Stay alert for "switchbacks". These are the words and phrases frequently used to alert you to shifts in thought. The most common switchback word is "but". Others include although, however, nevertheless, on the other hand, even though, while, in spite of, despite, regardless of.

Once you know which paragraph the answer will be in, focus on that paragraph. However, don't get distracted by a choice that is factually true about the paragraph. Your search is for the answer that answers the question, which may be about a tiny aspect in the paragraph. Stay focused and don't fall for an answer that describes the larger picture of the paragraph. Always go back to the question and make sure you're choosing an answer that actually answers the question and is not just a true statement.

The Science Reasoning Test

The Science Reasoning test may scare you. For even the most accomplished student, many of the terms will be unfamiliar. General test-taking skill will help the most. Make sure you don't run out of time: move quickly and use the easy pacing methods we outline in the test-taking tactics section.

The most important thing you can do is to ignore your fears and jump into the test immediately. Don't be overwhelmed by all of the strange-sounding terms. You have to jump into the test like jumping into a pool; all at once is the easiest way. Once you get past the jargon, you'll find that the Science Reasoning test is in some ways easier than even the Reading Test. Unfortunately, most students don't finish this test. This is why managing your time on this test is at least as important as on the Math test.

The test will have 7 sections. Each section is about the same difficulty. Some will be harder for you, of course, so let's plan ahead.

The test lasts 35 minutes, 5 minutes per section.

The first thing to do is to read the passage. Use 2 minutes to do this. Really try to understand what's going on, treating all of the scientific terms as you would characters in a novel; just accept their names as they are, and follow the story. Use another 3 minutes to answer as many questions as you can, then **move on to the next section**. It's important to answer all of the easy questions.

Overall, the Science Reasoning is the test that is hardest to study for has the lowest test average for all test-takers, even lower than the Math. If science is a subject you take because you have to, and not because you want to, your primary goal on Science Reasoning is damage control; you want to prevent it from dragging down your higher scores when ACT averages your test scores to get the composite.

In addition, the Science Reasoning test is probably unlike any other science test you've ever taken in high school. It's vital that you work a few practice Science Reasoning tests before the test day. Familiarity alone will boost your score by 1-2 points.

Four Types of Passages

Each of the seven sections in Science Reasoning has one of four possible types of passages:

1. Graph Mania: two or more graphs with questions about their meaning. You should start by asking yourself basic questions: *What are the variables? What are the units of measure? What are the values of the variables? What are the trends? What are the correlations?*

2. Table Mania: two or more tables containing data, with questions about their meaning. You should start by asking yourself basic questions: *What are the variables? What are the units of measure? What are the values of the variables? What are the trends? What are the correlations?*

3. Fighting Scientists: two different theories are explained for a natural process, and you answer questions about them. Short paragraphs will be provided representing the ideas of two scientists. They will disagree with each other. Your job is to analyze that argument and information in the two paragraphs. Approach it with the following questions: *What is the nature of the disagreement? How has the opinion been reached? What forms of evidence might resolve the conflict? What are the points of agreement and disagreement? What evidence supports or denies support for either viewpoint?*

4. Experiments: questions about data from experiments (usually two) performed. Experiment descriptions will be provided, along with a statement of the experiment's results. You should start by asking yourself basic questions: *What is the experiment designed to find out? What does the experimental method or any accompanying diagram reveal? What are the variables? What are the controls?* (Controls are precautions taken to eliminate all variables except the independent variable.) *What are the results?* Look for flaws in the experiment. *Are the controls adequate? Is the conclusion justified by the data? Are the experimental errors so great as to invalidate the results?* Once you thoroughly understand the nature of the experiment and the meaning of the results, you should be able to deal with the multiple-choice questions based on the experiment.

Four Types of Questions

The questions on the Science Reasoning test will fall into one of four categories:

1. Fact: this type asks for a fact, usually some sort of number, based on the passage. For example: *What is the volume of the gas at 1 atmosphere?*

2. Graphs: this type asks you to pick between graphs that best represent something described in the question.

3. Short answer: this type asks for a short answer, either a word or phrase, which answers a question about the passage. This question is identified not by the length of the answers (though they are usually short), but by how much thought is in the answer choice. For example, answer choices like *Day 1 at 12:00 PM* would be short answers. These kinds of questions are still asking for a simple fact.

4. Long answer: this type is an interpretation question about the passage that requires you to choose between several possible extended answers.

There are three question difficulty levels: understanding, analysis, and generalization. In each group of questions, the first ones will be understanding, and then will come the analysis questions, and finally the generalization questions. These are in increasing levels of difficulty as the earlier questions ask easy-to-find answers, while the later questions involve greater depth of interpretation and the ability to draw conclusions from the data.

Answer Choice Elimination Techniques

Informal Language
Answers that use formal or scientific language are better than ones that use informal language. In the answer choices below, choice *B* is much less formal and is incorrect, while choice *A* is a scientific, analytical choice and is correct.

Example:
  A. To compare the outcomes of the two different kinds of treatment.
  B. Because some subjects insisted on getting one or the other of the treatments.

Extreme Statements
Avoid answers that throw out highly controversial ideas that are proclaimed as established fact. In the example below, *A* is a radical idea and is most likely incorrect. *B* is a calm rational statement; it's most likely the correct answer. Notice that *B* does not make a definitive, uncompromising stance; it uses the hedge word *if* to provide wiggle room.

Example:
  A. Bypass surgery should be discontinued completely.
  B. Medication should be used instead of surgery for patients who have not had a heart attack if they suffer from mild chest pain and mild coronary artery blockage.

Similar Answer Choices

When you have two answer choices that are direct opposites, one of them is usually the correct answer.

Example:
- A. The effectiveness of enzyme I at 30 degrees Celsius depends on its concentration.
- B. The effectiveness of enzyme II at 30 degrees Celsius depends on its concentration.

These two answer choices are very similar and fall into the same family of answer choices. A family of answer choices is when two or three answer choices are very similar. Often two will be opposites and one may show an equality of some kind.

Example:
- A. Operation I or Operation II can be conducted at equal cost
- B. Operation I would be less expensive than Operation II
- C. Operation II would be less expensive than Operation I
- D. Neither Operation I nor Operation II would be effective at preventing the spread of cancer.

Note how the first three choices are all related. They all ask about a cost comparison. Beware of immediately recognizing B and C as opposites and choosing one of those two. A is in the same family of answers and should be considered as well. However, D is not in the same family of answers. It has nothing to do with cost and can be discounted in most cases.

Related to the family of answers concept are answer choices that have similar parts.

Example:
- A. The first stage of reaction 1 and the first stage of reaction 2.
- B. The second stage of reaction 1 and the second stage of reaction 3.
- C. The second stage of reaction 1 and the second stage of reaction 2.
- D. The second stage of reaction 1 and the first stage of reaction 2.

In this question, B, C, and D all begin with the same phrase *the second stage of reaction 1*. This means A can be eliminated. Then A and D both have the same phrase *the first stage of reaction 2*. Also, B and C have different phrases. This means that either A or D is the correct answer. Since A has already been eliminated, D is probably the right answer. In these cases similar phrases identify answer choices as being members of the same family of answers. Each answer choice that has a similar phrase is in the same family of answers. The answer choice that falls into the most family of answers is usually the correct answer.

Once again, hedge words are usually good, while answer choices without hedge words are typically wrong. Likewise, answer choices that use words like *exactly, never,* or *always* are usually wrong.

Time Management

Scan the passage to get a rough idea of what it is asking. Avoid answers that are obviously true but don't actually answer the question. Your choice must **answer** the question, not just be a factually true statement. The answer choice must be based strictly on the contents of the passage and question.

Read all the choices. Later answer choices will often bring up a new point that you may not have considered. As you read the choices, scratch through the ones that you know are wrong, but don't make your final selection until you read them all.

The easier understanding questions are listed first. Do not skip these first questions in each group, though everywhere else (on other tests and in other questions in the science test that aren't the first question in a group) you *should* skip questions that are giving you too much difficulty. This is because if you don't understand the passage, you're in real trouble on these harder questions. Make sure you know enough to get the first question right, because the other questions will all flow from a basic understanding of the passage. Skip the hard questions that aren't the first question in a group.

If the answers are numerical, estimate. Calculation takes time, and you should avoid it whenever possible. You can usually eliminate three obviously wrong choices quite easily.

For example, suppose a graph shows that an object has traveled 48 meters in 11 seconds, and you are asked to find its speed. You are given these choices:
A. 250 m/s
B. 42 m/s
C. 4.4 m/s
D. 1.2 m/s

You know that 48 divided by 11 will be a little over 4, so you can pick out *C* as the answer without ever doing the calculation.

Highly Technical Questions May Not Be

Sometimes a single piece of information may be given to you. For example: *Blood velocity is lowest in the capillaries (averaging 3cm/sec)*. A question may ask the following:

A physician examining a newly discovered tribe of people deep in the Amazon jungles found that the relative total surface area of their capillaries was greater than that previously reported for any other people. If the physician were to predict the average velocity of blood through their capillaries, which of the following values would be the most reasonable.
A. 2 cm/sec
B. 3 cm/sec
C. 4 cm/sec
D. 5 cm/sec

You know that 3 cm/sec is the standard, which is *B*. Without understanding any of the subject matter or even reading the associated graph, it is possible to choose the correct answer, which is *A*. The reason is because there is only one answer which is less than 3 cm/sec, while there are two answers that are greater than 3 cm/sec. Since you are not looking for an exact answer, but only a reasonable answer, then you can conclude that if the correct answer were greater than 3 cm/sec, two answer choices would meet that criterion. However, if the correct answer is less than 3 cm/sec, only one answer choice meets that criteria, meaning it is likely the correct answer.

Experiment Passages

The best way to remember three different but similar experiments is to focus on the differences between the experiments. Between the first and second experiment, what was changed? Between the second and third experiment, what was done differently? That will keep the overall experiments properly aligned in your mind,

Random Tips

- On fact questions that require choosing between numbers, don't guess the smallest or largest choice unless you're sure of the answer (remember, *sure* means you would bet $5 on it).
- Short answer questions want you to choose between several words that are choices. Your best weapon on these is process of elimination. There are no easy tips.
- The long answer questions will often have a few "bizarre" choices, mentioning things that are not relevant to the passage. Also, avoid answers that sound highly "intellectual." Again, if you're willing to bet $5, disregard the tips and go with your bet.
- In passages that describe a series of experiments, often the questions will ask you if the researcher made a mistake, or could improve the experiments by making some change; the answer choices will be two *yes's* and two *no's*, each with a different justification. Usually, the answer is one of the *no* choices. The ACT does not include deliberately flawed experiments in passages, so it is safe to assume that whatever suggestion the question poses would *not* improve the experiment. Keep in mind that *usually* does not mean *always*, so if you're sure that the answer is *no* ($5 confidence), disregard the tip.
- This bears repeating, especially on this test: you have probably never had a science test quite like the ACT Science Reasoning. You *must* take at least one practice test so as to not be bogged down with the unfamiliar format.

The Writing Test

A topic will be presented to you and you must write out a discussion on it within the 30 minutes allowed. There is not a "correct" answer to the topic. You must evaluate the topic, organize your ideas, and develop them into a cohesive and coherent response.

You will be scored on how well you are able to utilize standard written English, organize and explain your thoughts, and support those thoughts with reasons and examples.

Brainstorm

Spend the first three to five minutes brainstorming out ideas. Write down any ideas you might have on the topic. The purpose is to extract from the recesses of your memory any relevant information. In this stage, anything goes down. Write down any idea, regardless of how good it may initially seem. You can use either the scratch paper provided or the word processor to quickly jot down your thoughts and ideas. The word processor is highly recommended though, particularly if you are a fast typist.

Strength through Diversity

The best papers will contain diversity of examples and reasoning. As you brainstorm consider different perspectives. Not only are there two sides to every issue, but there are also countless perspectives that can be considered. On any issue, different groups are impacted, with many reaching the same conclusion or position, but through vastly different paths. Try to "see" the issue through as many different eyes as you can. Look at it from every angle and from every vantage point. The more diverse the reasoning used, the more balanced the paper will become and the better the score.

Example: The issue of free trade is not just two sided. It impacts politicians, domestic (US) manufacturers, foreign manufacturers, the US economy, the world economy, strategic alliances, retailers, wholesalers, consumers, unions, workers, and the exchange of more than just goods, but also of ideas, beliefs, and cultures. The more of these angles that you can approach the issue from, the more solid your reasoning and the stronger your position.

Furthermore, don't just use information as to how the issue impacts other people. Draw liberally from your own experience and your own observations. Explain a personal experience that you have had and your own emotions from that moment. Anything that you've seen in your community or observed in society can be expanded upon to further round out your position on the issue.

Pick a Main Idea

Once you have finished with your creative flow, stop and review it. Which idea were you able to come up with the most supporting information? It's extremely important that you pick an angle that will allow you to have a thorough and comprehensive coverage of the topic. This is not about your personal convictions, but about writing a concise rational discussion of an idea.

Weed the Garden

Every garden of ideas gets weeds in it. The ideas that you brainstormed over are going to be random pieces of information of mixed value. Go through it methodically and pick out the ones that are the best. The best ideas are strong points that it will be easy to write a few sentences or a paragraph about.

Create a Logical Flow

Now that you know which ideas you are going to use and focus upon, organize them. Put your writing points in a logical order. You have your main ideas that you will focus on, and must align them in a sequence that will flow in a smooth, sensible path from point to point, so that the reader will go smoothly from one idea to the next in a logical path. Readers must have a sense of continuity as they read your paper. You don't want to have a paper that rambles back and forth.

Start Your Engines

You have a logical flow of main ideas with which to start writing. Begin expanding on the issues in the sequence that you have set for yourself. Pace yourself. Don't spend too much time on any one of the ideas that you are expanding upon. You want to have time for all of them. Make sure you watch your time. If you have twenty minutes left to write out your ideas and you have ten ideas, then you can only use two minutes per idea. It can be a daunting task to cram a lot of information down in words in a short amount of time, but if you pace yourself, you can get through it all. If you find that you are falling behind, speed up. Move through each idea more quickly, spending less time to expand upon the idea in order to catch back up.

Once you finish expanding on each idea, go back to your brainstorming session up above, where you wrote out your ideas. Go ahead and erase the ideas as you write about them. This will let you see what you need to write about next, and also allow you to pace yourself and see what you have left to cover.

First Paragraph

Your first paragraph should have several easily identifiable features.
- First, it should have a quick description or paraphrasing of the topic. Use your own words to briefly explain what the topic is about.
- Second, you should explain your opinion of the topic and give an explanation of why you feel that way. What is your decision or conclusion on the topic?
- Third, you should list your "writing points". What are the main ideas that you came up with earlier? This is your opportunity to outline the rest of your paper. Have a sentence explaining each idea that you will go intend further depth in additional paragraphs. If someone was to only read this paragraph, they should be able to get an "executive summary" of the entire paper.

Body Paragraph

Each of your successive paragraphs should expand upon one of the points listed in the main paragraph. Use your personal experience and knowledge to support each of your points. Examples should back up everything.

Conclusion Paragraph

Once you have finished expanding upon each of your main points, wrap it up. Summarize what you have said and covered in a conclusion paragraph. Explain once more your opinion of the topic and quickly review why you feel that way. At this stage, you have already backed up your statements, so there is no need to do that again. All you are doing is refreshing in the mind of the reader the main points that you have made.

Don't Panic

Panicking will not put down any more words on paper for you. Therefore, it isn't helpful. When you first see the topic, if your mind goes as blank as the page on which you have to write out your paper, take a deep breath. Force yourself to mechanically go through the steps listed above.

Secondly, don't get clock fever. It's easy to be overwhelmed when you're looking at a page that doesn't seem to have much text, there is a lot of blank space further down, your mind is full of random thoughts and feeling confused, and the clock is ticking down faster than you would like. You brainstormed first so that you don't have to keep coming up with ideas. If you're running out of time and you have a lot of ideas that you haven't expanded upon, don't be afraid to make some cuts. Start picking the best ideas that you have left and expand on those few. Don't feel like you have to write down and expand all of your ideas.

Check Your Work

It is more important to have a shorter paper that is well written and well organized, than a longer paper that is poorly written and poorly organized. Don't keep writing about a subject just to add words and sentences, and certainly don't start repeating yourself. Expand on the ideas that you identified in the brainstorming session and make sure that you save yourself a few minutes at the end to go back and check your work.

Leave time at the end, at least three minutes, to go back and check over your work. Reread and make sure that everything you've written makes sense and flows. Clean up any spelling or grammar mistakes that you might have made. If you see anything that needs to be moved around, such as a paragraph that would fit in better somewhere else, cut and paste it to that new location. Also, go ahead and erase any brainstorming ideas that you weren't able to expand upon and clean up any other extraneous information that you might have written that doesn't fit into your paper.

As you proofread, make sure there aren't any fragments or run-ons. Check for sentences that are too short or too long. If the sentence is too short, look to see if you have an identifiable subject and verb. If it is too long, break it up into two separate sentences. Watch out for any "big" words you may have used. It's good to use difficult vocabulary words, but only if you are positive that you are using them correctly. Your paper has to be correct, it doesn't have to be fancy. You're not trying to impress anyone with your vocabulary, just your ability to develop and express ideas.

Final Note

Depending on your test taking preferences and personality, the essay writing will probably be your hardest or your easiest section. You are required to go through the entire process of writing a paper in 30 minutes or less, which can be quite a challenge.

Focus upon each of the steps listed above. Go through the process of creative flow first, generating ideas and thoughts about the topic. Then organize those ideas into a smooth logical flow. Pick out the ones that are best from the list you have created. Decide which main idea or angle of the topic you will discuss.

Create a recognizable structure in your paper, with an introductory paragraph explaining what you have decided upon, and what your main points will be. Use the body paragraphs to expand on those main points and have a conclusion that wraps up the issue or topic.

Save a few moments to go back and review what you have written. Clean up any minor mistakes that you might have had and give it those last few critical touches that can make a huge difference. Finally, be proud and confident of what you have written!

Appendix A: Time Statistics for the ACT

ACT Time Constraints				
	English	Math	Reading	Science
Passages	5	N/A	4	7
Questions	75	60	40	40
Time (in minutes)	45	60	35	35
Questions/Passage	15	N/A	10	5.7
seconds/question	36	60	52.5	52.5
min/passage	9	N/A	8.75	5
words/passage	260	N/A	780	350
words/question	43	N/A	43	52
Reading rate (WPM)	200	200	200	200
Time used for passages (min)	7.5	N/A	12	14
Time left for questions	30	N/A	34.5	31.5

Appendix B: SAT/ACT Equivalency Table

ACT Composite Score	Recentered SAT I Score Verbal+Math
36	1600
35	1580
34	1520
33	1470
32	1420
31	1380
30	1340
29	1300
28	1260
27	1220
26	1180
25	1140
24	1110
23	1070
22	1030
21	990
20	950
19	910
18	870
17	830
16	780
15	740
14	680
13	620
12	560
11	500

Appendix C: Area, Volume, Surface Area Formulas

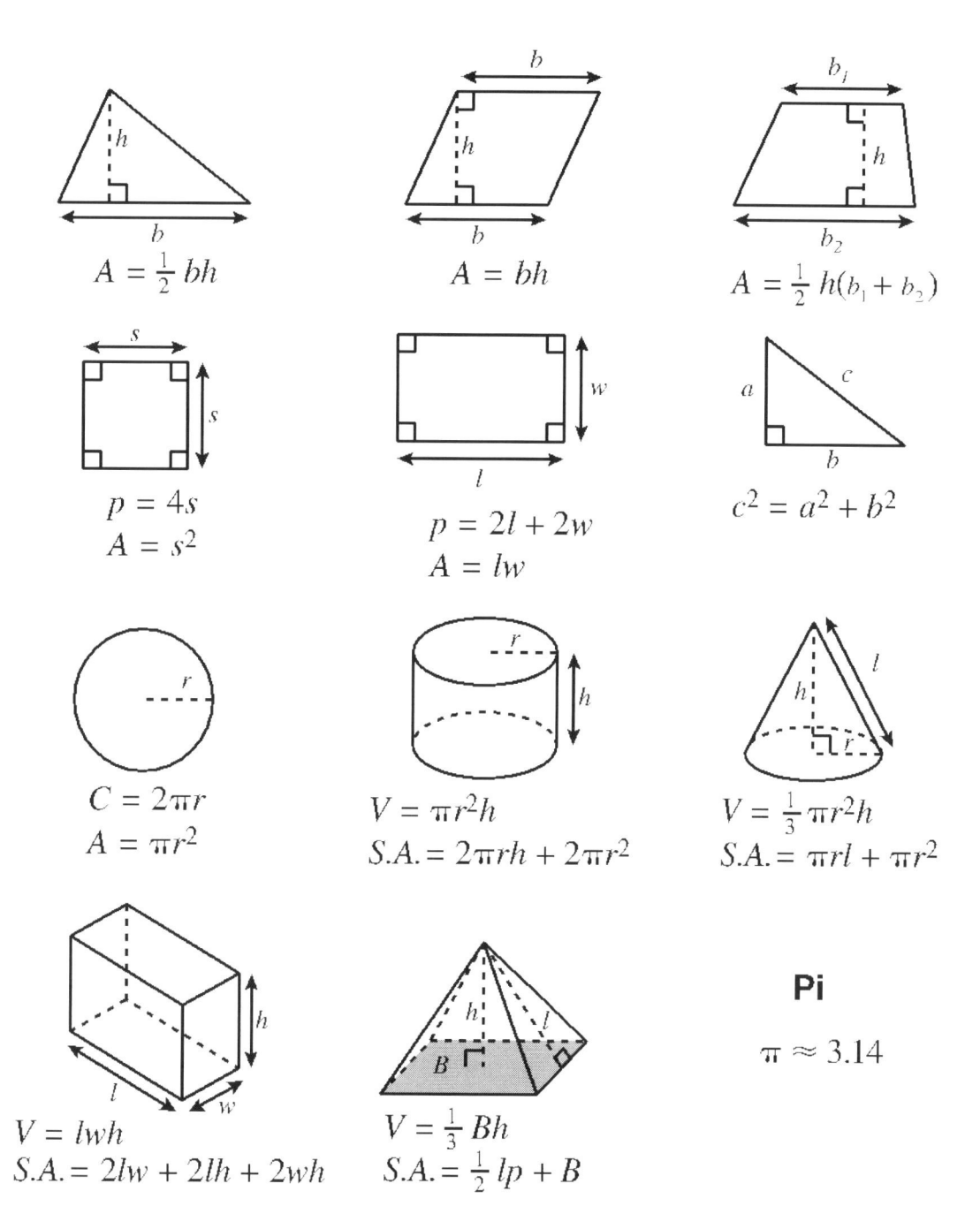

$A = \frac{1}{2} bh$

$A = bh$

$A = \frac{1}{2} h(b_1 + b_2)$

$p = 4s$
$A = s^2$

$p = 2l + 2w$
$A = lw$

$c^2 = a^2 + b^2$

$C = 2\pi r$
$A = \pi r^2$

$V = \pi r^2 h$
$S.A. = 2\pi rh + 2\pi r^2$

$V = \frac{1}{3} \pi r^2 h$
$S.A. = \pi rl + \pi r^2$

$V = lwh$
$S.A. = 2lw + 2lh + 2wh$

$V = \frac{1}{3} Bh$
$S.A. = \frac{1}{2} lp + B$

Pi

$\pi \approx 3.14$

Appendix D: Practice Test

English

Numbers 1-15 pertain to the following passage:

<u>Restoration of the Sistine Chapel</u>
The Sistine chapel holds a magnificent collection of Renaissance frescoes. The restoration of these frescoes (1) <u>is an important 20th century event</u> in the art world.

Completed in about 1481, (2) <u>the chapels' walls</u> were decorated by important Renaissance painters including Perugino and Botticelli. The paintings done in the 1500s by Michelangelo enhanced the artistic magnificence of the chapel.

The most recent restoration, begun in 1980, (3) <u>were preceded</u> by numerous restoration attempts. Records indicate that damage to the ceiling was noted as early as 1547. Restoration attempts in 1625, early 1700s, and the 1930s attempted (4) <u>to restore and maintaining</u> the original beauty of the artworks.

The modern restoration began in 1979 (5) <u>with study and analysis</u> of the artwork; this investigation into the composition and condition of the works lasted six months. The team's mandate (6) <u>including</u> recording every step of the restoration, repairing structural damage, and using only materials and procedures that were not harmful and were (7) <u>reversible.</u>

The restorers' analysis revealed that the entire chapel was covered with candle smoke and that the building was unstable and had shifted, causing cracking (8) <u>in the ceiling.</u> (9) <u>In additionally,</u> water seepage from the roof carried salts down and deposited them on the ceiling. Early restorations had also done some damage: the materials early restorers had used (animal fat and vegetable oil) left a (10) <u>sticky-dirty</u> and filmy layer on the frescoes.

The restoration (11) <u>spark</u> controversy even before it was begun. Concerns (12) <u>are voiced</u> about the possibility of damage to the artwork (13) <u>from a result</u> of the restoration; critics noted that damage had been done during every other restoration attempt. The area of greatest concern was (14) <u>Michelangelos'</u> ceiling. The restorers made a decision that Michelangelo painted in a particular manner throughout the artwork, and thus treated the entire ceiling the same in their restoration efforts. The critics argue that this assumption (15) <u>is too broadly</u> and that damage was done by the restoration approach. The critics also argue that what the restorers treated as soot that should be removed, was actually paint used by Michelangelo to provide shadows and definition. In addition, the cleaning involved in the restoration removed the eyes from numerous figures.

1. A. no change
   B. was important 20th century events
   C. was an important 20th century event
   D. were an important 20th century event

2. F. no change
   G. the chapel's walls
   H. the chapel's wall
   J. the chapels walls

3. A. no change
   B. is preceded
   C. been preceded
   D. was preceded

4. F. no change
   G. to restoring and maintaining
   H. to restoring and maintain
   J. to restore and maintain

5. A. no change
   B. on study and analysis
   C. because study and analysis
   D. upon study and analysis

6. F. no change
   G. included
   H. include
   J. includes

7. A. no change
   B. reversing
   C. reversibly
   D. reverse

8. F. no change
   G. above the ceiling
   H. without the ceiling
   J. before the ceiling

9. A. no change
   B. In addition,
   C. Addition,
   D. In additional,

10. F. no change
    G. sticky plus dirty
    H. sticky, dirty
    J. sticky-dirt

11. A. no change
    B. sparked
    C. sparking
    D. sparkedly

12. F. no change
    G. is voiced
    H. voicing
    J. were voiced

13. A. no change
    B. as a result
    C. in a result
    D. of a result

14. F. no change
    G. Michelangelo's
    H. Michelangelo
    J. Michelangelos

15. A. no change
    B. is broadly
    C. broadly
    D. is too broad

Numbers 16-30 pertain to the following passage:

A Quick (and Easy) Step to Better Health

A more healthy diet is something most of us want. It can be mystifying to put into practice sometimes though – with new (and completely different) diet books coming (16) of the market every day that tell us that if we follow them (17) precise they will not only make us thinner, but stronger, smarter and help us live longer. Sometimes it's easier to just throw up our hands and eat that bag of Cheetos for dinner, than (18) to decide how we're going to make sense of all the eating advice out there. Just because it's hard and frustrating doesn't mean (19) its okay to stop trying (20) through. Endless snacking on those Cheetos may be understandable if we can't figure out exactly how to do things right, but it's also a sure-fire way to be a whole lot less healthy if it keeps us from eating better options.

One powerful (21) but very easily approach to increasing the healthiness of our diets is to recognize that some foods are so good for us that we can almost think of them as medicine. Some fight heart disease or cancer, some lower cholesterol or blood pressure. Some fight depression. At some point, (22) we may wants to give ourselves the complete diet, exercise, and general health overhaul that all these books seem to think is necessary, but (23) in the meantime, we can take the baby step of adding in one or more good-for-us foods a week. This step is quick, easy, painless and couldn't be simpler (24) implement—and it will make our transition to full-fledged healthy eating that much easier to accomplish when we finally get there.

Here are a few ideas for superstar foods to work in to our regular diet: broccoli has tons of vitamin K and vitamin C which help build strong bones and fight off cancers. Dark chocolate can (25) reducing blood pressure as well as bad cholesterol. Walnuts and salmon have tons of omega-3 fatty acids which are linked to reduced risk of depression, heart disease and cancer. Lemons pack in the vitamin C, may inhibit the growth of cancer cells and (26) acts as an anti-inflammatory. Avocadoes can lower cholesterol and help reduce risk of heart disease. Sweet potatoes are jam-packed full of cancer-fighting and immune system-boosting vitamin A. Garlic can inhibit the growth of bacteria and has been shown to lower cholesterol and blood pressure. Spinach is a great cancer fighter and contains immune-boosting antioxidants important for eye health. Beans help lower risk of heart disease and breast cancer.

Wouldn't we take all (27) that things if they were medicines that our doctors offered us? Instead, we have the fun (28) off sitting back with (29) our lemony guacamole, bean salad, grilled salmon or piece of dark chocolate and knowing we're taking an important (30) steps to better health.

16. F. no change
    G. on the market
    H. from the market
    J. if the market

17. A. no change
    B. precision
    C. precisefully
    D. precisely

18. F. no change
    G. decided
    H. deciding
    J. make decision

19. A. no change
    B. it are
    C. it's
    D. all

20. F. no change
    G. though
    H. thus
    J. throughout

21. A. no change
    B. but very easy
    C. but not easy
    D. but not easily

22. F. no change
    G. we may
    H. we wants
    J. we may want

23. A. no change
    B. in the now
    C. in the time now
    D. in meantime

24. F. no change
    G. implementing
    H. implementation
    J. to implement

25. A. no change
    B. reduce
    C. reduction
    D. reduces

26. F. no change
    G. act on
    H. act
    J. acting

27. A. no change
    B. this things
    C. these things
    D. that

28. F. no change
    G. and
    H. around
    J. of

29. A. no change
    B. his
    C. her
    D. my

30. F. no change
    G. step
    H. stepping
    J. step on

Numbers 31-45 pertain to the following passage:

Medical Errors

In the United States, medical errors (inaccurate diagnoses or treatment) (31) are estimate to result in 44,000 to 98,000 unnecessary deaths, and 1 million unnecessary injuries (32) each years. Errors can include misdiagnosis, administration of the wrong drug, surgery on the wrong site (E.G., the wrong limb), among others.

Medical errors have many (33) sources: inexperienced doctors or other medical staff, poor doctor-patient communication, sleep deprivation of medical staff, poor documentation, inadequate staffing and similarly named medications. (34) A significant numbers of medical errors occur in the diagnosis of psychological disorders.

One study found that being awake for over 24 hours caused medical interns to (35) more than doubling the number of preventable medical errors they made. U.S. federal regulations do not limit the (36) number of hour that can be assigned during a graduate medical (37) student's medical residency. Residents routinely work close to 100 hours a week and surgical residents often work (38) even as much than that.

(39) In the past: most doctors did not acknowledge errors (40) they had commit, causing a general lack of patient trust. In 2007, 34 (41) states passes legislation precluding information from a physician's apology from (42) being used in a malpractice suit. This protection makes doctors (43) comfortabler acknowledging and explaining errors (44) at patients and the current practice is (45) to disclose errors as soon as they are noticed.

31. A. no change
    B. estimate
    C. estimating
    D. are estimated

72

32. F. no change
    G. each year
    H. all years
    J. each yearly

33. A. no change
    B. sources. Inexperienced
    C. sources inexperienced
    D. sources? Inexperienced

34. F. no change
    G. Significant number
    H. A significant number
    J. Significant numerous

35. A. no change
    B. more than doubles
    C. more than double
    D. more double

36. F. no change
    G. numbers of hour
    H. hour number
    J. number of hours

37. A. no change
    B. students'
    C. student
    D. student'

38. F. no change
    G. even more than
    H. even so many as
    J. even up to more

39. A. no change
    B. In the past, most
    C. In the past most
    D. In the past; most

40. F. no change
    G. they commit
    H. they commits
    J. they had committed

41. A. no change
    B. states passed
    C. states' passed
    D. state's passed

42. F. no change
    G. being use
    H. being useful
    J. being

43. A. no change
    B. comfortablest
    C. more comfortabler
    D. more comfortable

44. F. no change
    G. to patients
    H. on patients
    J. in patients

45. A. no change
    B. disclosing errors
    C. disclosed errors
    D. discloses errors

Numbers 46-60 pertain to the following passage:

H.M.S. Pinafore

An (46) <u>international</u> famous Gilbert and Sullivan comic opera, the H.M.S Pinafore, tells the story of life (47) <u>above</u> the ship of the title, the H.M.S. Pinafore. (48) <u>Josephine - the</u> captain's daughter, is expected to marry the First Lord of the Admiralty, Sir Joseph, but is (49) <u>inconveniently</u> in love with a lower-class sailor, Ralph Rackstraw.

Josephine accepts her intended future (50) <u>at firstly</u> but after Rackstraw (51) <u>heres</u> Sir Joseph advocate equality of all people, he decides (52) <u>declare</u> his love to Josephine and she decides (53) <u>to elope</u> with Rackstraw. Much conflict and confusion arise, but ultimately a surprise twist reveals that the Captain and Rackstraw (54) <u>are switched</u> as babies so the Captain, and Josephine, are in fact lower class and Rackstraw belongs to the higher social class. Sir Joseph (55) <u>now longer</u> wants to marry Josephine, who then happily marries Rackstraw.

The (56) <u>operas'</u> extraordinary worldwide success paved the way for the continued phenomenal success of additional Gilbert and Sullivan works. These works (57) <u>dominate</u> the musical stage for more than ten years and are still performed today.

Gilbert began work on Pinafore in 1877. Sullivan finalized the music in 1878. Pinafore opened on May 25, 1878 at the Opera Cacique. Initial reviews of Pinafore were (58) <u>mostly favoring.</u> Modern American productions (59) <u>continued to this day</u> to be generally well-received. Since the copyright expiration of the opera, companies around the world have been free to produce, (60) <u>and freely adapt,</u> Gilbert and Sullivan works.

46. F. no change
    G. internation
    H. internationally
    J. internet

47. A. no change
    B. in
    C. with
    D. on

48. F. no change
    G. Josephine, the
    H. Josephine (the
    J. Josephine the

49. A. no change
    B. inconvenience
    C. inconvene
    D. convenience

50. F. no change
    G. at fist
    H. firstly
    J. at first

51. A. no change
    B. hares
    C. hears
    D. here's

52. F. no change
    G. declaring
    H. to declare
    J. declares

53. A. no change
    B. elope
    C. eloping
    D. to elopes

54. F. no change
    G. were switched
    H. are switching
    J. are switch

55. A. no change
    B. now long
    C. no longer
    D. no long

56. F. no change
    G. opera's
    H. operas
    J. opera

57. A. no change
    B. dominates
    C. dominated
    D. dominator

58. F. no change
    G. mostly favorable
    H. most favorable
    J. more favorable

59. A. no change
    B. continue
    C. continuing
    D. continues

60. F. no change
    G. and freely adapting
    H. and freely adapt on
    J. and freely adapts

Numbers 61-75 pertain to the following passage:

Shotgun Houses

> The following paragraphs may or may not be in the most logical order. You may be asked questions about the logical order of the paragraphs, as well as where to place sentences logically within any given paragraph.

A shotgun house is a (61) narrow usually no more than 12 feet wide - rectangular home with doors at each end. The houses consist of between three and five rooms, all lined in a row with no hallways. Typically the living room is the first room, followed by one or two bedrooms and a kitchen in the back. Early shotgun houses were built without a bathroom. The name is often said to come from the idea that one could fire a shotgun through the front door clean through the back door.

Shotgun houses are almost always (62) closer to the street with a small, if any, front yard. The house is usually raised a couple feet off the ground. Originally doors and windows would have been covered by decorative shutters. Typically the houses were wood frame structure with wood siding. Rooms are well-sized with high ceilings to allow the heat to rise.

The shotgun house (63) was the most popular style of house in the U.S. South from the end of the Civil War until the 1920s. It was developed in New Orleans, but the style spread and shotgun houses can be found in many far-flung places including Illinois, Florida and California. The shotgun style became so popular in part because, prior to widespread car ownership, people working in urban areas (64) needed to live close to city centers. Shotgun houses were often initially built as rental properties to provide housing for manufacturing or railroad workers. Factory owners often built the houses specifically to rent to their employees. By the late 20th century, shotguns were often owner occupied.

(65) Another advantages to the shotgun style is the fact that its length contributed to good airflow – an (68) important factor in hot urban areas of the South. Shotgun house building lots were small, which allowed the high demand for city housing to be met.

The construction of shotgun houses (69) slowing and then stopped entirely during the early 20th century (70) after the advent of the car and indoor air conditioning. From World War II until the 1980s, (71) people seen shotguns as substandard housing and a symbol of poverty. Many were demolished as part of urban renewal projects.

Many neighborhoods in southern American cities (72) <u>still contains</u> a large number of shotgun houses. New Orleans, Louisville and Atlanta (73) <u>each</u> have neighborhoods with high shotgun house concentrations. The homes are also part of our idea of life in the southern: Elvis Presley was born in a shotgun house, the (74) <u>Neville Brothers grow up</u> in one and (75) <u>legend has it</u> that Robert Johnson died in one.

61. A. no change
    B. narrow – usually
    C. narrow, usually
    D. narrow (usually

62. F. no change
    G. close
    H. closing
    J. closest

63. A. no change
    B. were
    C. is
    D. has

64. F. no change
    G. needs to live
    H. need to live
    J. need to living

65. A. no change
    B. Another advantageous
    C. Another advantages
    D. Another advantage

66. Which of the following choices improves the fourth paragraph?
    F. no change
    G. Changing the order of the two sentences.
    H. Eliminating the phrase "an important factor in hot urban areas of the South."
    J. Changing the word "contributed" to "generated."

67. The following sentence would most appropriately be placed at the end of which paragraph?

    Thus, even if many end up demolished, shotgun houses will remain forever part of the Unites States' architectural history and cultural memory.

    A. third
    B. fourth
    C. fifth
    D. sixth

68. F. no change
    G. important fact
    H. important faction
    J. import factor

69. A. no change
    B. slows
    C. slow
    D. slowed

70. F. no change
    G. after advent
    H. preceding the advent
    J. despite the advent

71. A. no change
    B. people see
    C. people saw
    D. people seer

72. F. no change
    G. still contain
    H. stills contain
    J. still containing

73. A. no change
    B. some
    C. few
    D. all

74. F. no change
    G. grown up
    H. grew up
    J. growing up

75. A. no change
    B. legend has
    C. legend have
    D. legend hasn't

Mathematics

1. Steven wants to put trim around the edge of a quilt that is 7 feet long by 6 feet wide. How much trim, in feet, does Steven need?
    A. 13
    B. 14
    C. 26
    D. 28
    E. 30

2. A teacher graded the first 5 tests in a stack. She gave a 76, 80, 69 and 71 for the first four tests. If she gave an average grade of 74 for the five tests, what grade did she give the fifth test?
    F. 74
    G. 75
    H. 76
    J. 77
    K. 79

3. Mary ate $1\frac{2}{3}$ cups of rice last week and 2 and $\frac{3}{7}$ cups of rice this week. How much rice total did she eat in those two weeks?
    A. $3\frac{5}{10}$
    B. $4\frac{5}{10}$
    C. $3\frac{2}{21}$
    D. $4\frac{2}{21}$
    E. $5\frac{2}{21}$

4. If 3x – 2 = 5x -14, then x equals:
    F. 3
    G. 6
    H. 9
    J. 12
    K. 14

5. Mathilda's new job comes with a salary increase of 8%. If she currently makes $64,000 per year, which of the following is closest to what she will earn per year at her new job?
    A. $69,000
    B. $70,000
    C. $71,000
    D. $72,000
    E. $76,000

6. If David biked 10 miles in 4 hours and Mary biked three times as much in half the time, what was Mary's average rate of speed?
    F. 5 mph
    G. 10 mph
    H. 15 mph
    J. 20 mph
    K. 25 mph

7. The expression (4x – 3)(x + 2) is equivalent to
    A. $4x^2 - x + 2$
    B. x - 6
    C. $4x^2 + 8x - 6$
    D. $4x^2 + 5x - 6$
    E. 4x - 6

8. $|-4|^2 + |-7| - 2 =$
    F. 21
    G. 13
    H. 7
    J. 25
    K. 17

9. A house is 45 feet wide and divided into two rooms. If one room is twice as wide as the other, how wide is the smaller room?
    A. 10 feet
    B. 15 feet
    C. 20 feet
    D. 30 feet
    E. 35 feet

10. Abe averages 3 miles per hour running and Beatriz averages 4 miles per hour running. How much further can Beatriz go in $\frac{1}{2}$ hour than Abe can?
    F. 2 miles
    G. 1 mile
    H. $\frac{1}{2}$ mile
    J. $\frac{1}{4}$ mile
    K. $\frac{1}{8}$ mile

11. The 5 consecutive integers below add up to 190. What is the value of x?
    x – 2
    x – 1
    x
    x + 1
    x + 2
    A. 38
    B. 37
    C. 36
    D. 35
    E. 34

12. What is the least common multiplier of 5, 4x, 6y and 3xy?
    F. 30xy
    G. 60xy
    H. $60(xy)^2$
    J. $72(xy)^2$
    K. 72xy

13. |8 - 7| – |7 - 8| =
    A. -1
    B. 0
    C. 1
    D. 2
    E. 3

14. The child care center charges $11 an hour plus a daily $3 drop-off fee. How many hours of childcare did Robert pay for if he dropped his son off 3 days last week and paid $130 at the end of the week?
    F. 5
    G. 7
    H. 9
    J. 11
    K. 13

15. If a = -2 and b = -4, then $a^2b + 2ab$ =
    A. 0
    B. 4
    C. 16
    D. 32
    E. 40

16. Anna walks from her house to school each day. If she walks 8 blocks east of her house, then turns and walks 6 blocks south to arrive at school, how far is her school in a direct line from her house?
    F. 10 blocks
    G. 12 blocks
    H. 14 blocks
    J. 16 blocks
    K. 18 blocks

17. The average of x and y is 7 and the average of x, y and z is 9. What is the value of z?
    A. 7
    B. 9
    C. 11
    D. 13
    E. 15

18. Allison spends $\frac{1}{10}$ of her salary on transportation costs. Of that $\frac{1}{10}$, 80% is spent on gas. If Allison spends $200 on gas a month, what is her annual salary?
    F. $2500
    G. $15,000
    H. $30,000
    J. $45,000
    K. $60,000

19. It took Alex 1 hour and 39 minutes to complete his math homework. If he completed 33 problems in that time, how long did it take him on average to complete each problem?
    A. 3 minutes
    B. 5 minutes
    C. 7 minutes
    D. 9 minutes
    E. 11 minutes

20. If |x| = x + 14, then x =
    F. 0
    G. 7
    H. -7
    J. -14
    K. 14

21. To be qualified for a certain job opening, applicants need to satisfactorily complete a written application and an oral exam. Historically, 65% of applicants passed the written exam step, and 40% of those then passed the oral exam. Based on those figures, approximately how many applicants of a pool of 100 would you expect to be qualified for the job?
    A. 65
    B. 40
    C. 26
    D. 13
    E. 7

Questions 22 and 23 refer to the following information:

   Raul, Eli, Henry and Lex all bought the same shirt from different stores for different prices. They spent $18.00, $18.50, $15.39 and $19.99 respectively.

22. What is the average price the four men spent for the shirt?
    F. $15.97
    G. $16.97
    H. $17.97
    J. $18.97
    K. $19.97

23. How much more did the man who spent the most for the shirt spend than the man who spent the least for the shirt?
    A. $2.60
    B. $3.60
    C. $4.60
    D. $5.60
    E. $6.60

24. If candy is sold per pound, and $\frac{3}{4}$ of a pound costs $5.25, approximately how much would $1\frac{2}{3}$ of a pound cost?
    F. $10.66
    G. $10.96
    H. $11.66
    J. $11.96
    K. $12.66

25. In a survey done by a local news station, 33 people were against the new library bond, 64 people were for it, and 13 people were undecided. How can the number of people opposed to the library bond be expressed as a fraction?
    A. $\frac{3}{10}$

    B. $\frac{33}{100}$

    C. $\frac{3}{5}$

    D. $\frac{13}{100}$

    E. $\frac{4}{5}$

26. If a plank 17 feet 8 inches long is cut into two equal pieces, how long is each of the two pieces?
    F. 7 feet 4 inches
    G. 7 feet 10 inches
    H. 8 feet 4 inches
    J. 8 feet 10 inches
    K. 9 feet 4 inches

27. If Fahrenheit and Celsius are related by the formula $F = (\frac{9}{5})C + 32$, what is the temperature in degrees Fahrenheit of a location with an average temperature of 20 degrees Celsius?
    A. 58
    B. 63
    C. 68
    D. 73
    E. 78

28. A rectangle with a perimeter of 92 inches has a length of 14 inches longer than its width. What is its width in inches?
    F. 8
    G. 16
    H. 32
    J. 40
    K. 44

29. To qualify for the advanced Spanish class, students need an average of 90% on the 3 tests in intermediate Spanish. If Roxy received a 78% on the first test and a 95% on the second, what is the minimum she needs to receive on the third to qualify?
    A. 83
    B. 87
    C. 93
    D. 97
    E. 99

30. Tia and her brother Eli loan each other money and who owes who is constantly changing. If Tia owed Eli $13 at the start of last week, and now Eli owes Tia $8, by how many dollars has Eli's debt to Tia changed in that time period?
    F. $21
    G. $19
    H. $15
    J. $5
    K. $3

31. Disregarding sales tax, approximately how much will Diane save when she buys a $49.95 shirt that is on sale for 15% off?
    A. $3.50
    B. $5.00
    C. $7.00
    D. $7.50
    E. $8.00

32. What is the cubic volume of a box whose edges each measure 6 inches in length?
    F. 36
    G. 64
    H. 106
    J. 216
    K. 240

Questions 33 - 35 refer to the following information:

The 180 campers in Group A got to choose which kind of sandwich they wanted on the picnic. The results of the choice are given in the table below.

Sandwich	# of Campers
PB & J	60
Turkey	45
Egg salad	15
Veggie	60

33. Approximately what percentage of the campers chose either turkey or egg salad?
    A. 66
    B. 45
    C. 33
    D. 15
    E. 7

34. If the choices made by Group A are indicative of how all the campers would choose, how many of the 420 campers in the entire camp would choose PB & J?
    F. 140
    G. 130
    H. 120
    J. 110
    K. 100

35. Which expression correctly provides the ratio of campers who chose veggie sandwiches to those who chose turkey?
    A. 1:4
    B. 2:3
    C. 1:3
    D. 4:3
    E. 3:2

36. What is the largest integer less than the square root of 71?
    F. 7
    G. 8
    H. 9
    J. 10
    K. 11

37. Sarah has a sticker book that has 8 pages. Each page has room for up to 4 stickers on it. If Sarah gets 16 stickers and puts at least one sticker on each page, what is the greatest number of pages that can be filled with stickers?
   A. 1
   B. 2
   C. 4
   D. 6
   E. 8

38. The 10-member drama club earned funds for their trip to New York by selling tickets to their play. If they sold a total of 61 tickets for $10 each and the trip to New York will cost each student $525, how much does each student still need to raise?
   F. 364
   G. 394
   H. 424
   J. 464
   K. 524

39. 17.361 x 0.001 = _____
   A. 0.17361
   B. 0.017361
   C. 0.0017361
   D. 0.00017361
   E. 0.000017361

40. Charlie gets an allowance of $10 a week plus 75 cents for every additional chore he completes. If he received $13.75 last week, how many additional chores did he complete that week?
   F. 2
   G. 3
   H. 4
   J. 5
   K. 6

41. If 14 − x = 73, then x = _____
   A. 59
   B. 39
   C. -39
   D. -59
   E. 49

42. Sophie is painting a wall in her living room red She can cover 36 square feet with one gallon of paint. If the wall is 8 feet high and 15 feet long, how many gallons, to the nearest gallon, does she need?
   F. 2
   G. 3
   H. 4
   J. 5
   K. 6

43. What is $\frac{1}{2}$ of 18% of $36,000?
    A. 3,240
    B. 6,480
    C. 7,360
    D. 9,840
    E. 11,260

44. If 3x – 2 = 5x -12, x = _____
    F. 10
    G. 5
    H. 3
    J. 2
    K. 1

45. Which of the following is an equivalent form of 2x + x (x + x + x + x) – x?
    A. $x^2 + 4x$
    B. $4x^2 + x$
    C. $8x^2 + x$
    D. $4x^2 - x$
    E. 8x

Questions 46 – 47 refer to the following information:

Assume the statements below are true:
- Everyone who lives on Elm Street has a green front lawn
- Ashton has a green front lawn
- Elizabeth has a fig tree
- Trina lives on Elm Street
- Clara doesn't have a lawn
- Peter has a flower bed
- Gabriel has a lawn in his back yard

46. Considering only the statements above, which of the following must be false?
    F. Ashton lives on Elm Street
    G. Elizabeth lives on Elm Street
    H. Clara lives on Elm Street
    J. Peter lives on Elm Street
    K. Gabriel lives on Elm Street

47. Considering only the statements above, which of the following must be true?
    A. Peter and Ashton are not next door neighbors.
    B. Clara and Trina are not next door neighbors.
    C. Elizabeth and Trina are not next door neighbors.
    D. Elizabeth and Gabriel are not next door neighbors.
    E. Peter and Gabriel are not next door neighbors.

48. If y = 4, what is the value of x if $y^2 - 2y - x = 0$?
    F. 8
    G. 9
    H. 12
    J. 16
    K. 18

49. An organization's membership tripled during the year. At the end of the year, after the membership had tripled, half the membership left to form a splinter organization. If the remaining membership after the splinter group left was 75, what was the membership before it tripled?
    A. 100
    B. 80
    C. 50
    D. 30
    E. 20

50. Zachary has enough rope to reach 40 feet. If he uses the rope to enclose a square area, how many square feet will he enclose?
    F. 40
    G. 60
    H. 80
    J. 100
    K. 120

51. |7 - 4| – |1 - 7| =
    A. -5
    B. -3
    C. 3
    D. 5
    E. -1

52. Eli and Melanie bought some sandwiches and some drinks. Eli paid $8.00 for two sandwiches and six drinks. Melanie paid $8.00 for three sandwiches and one drink. What is the price of one sandwich?
    F. $1.50
    G. $2.00
    H. $2.50
    J. $3.00
    K. $3.50

53. From every three bananas he has, Ian can make one loaf of banana bread. If he has 8 bananas and makes all the loaves he can make from them, how many bananas will he have left over?
    A. 1
    B. 2
    C. 3
    D. 4
    E. 5

54. James won a cash raffle prize. He paid taxes of 30% on the prize and had $14,000 remaining. How much was the original prize?
    F. $42,000
    G. $40,000
    H. $30,000
    J. $20,000
    K. $18,000

55. What is the absolute value of 7 – x if x is 13?
    A. 6
    B. -6
    C. 8
    D. -8
    E. 20

56. The average of 5 consecutive numbers is 9. What is the sum of the least and the greatest of the numbers?
    F. 7
    G. 11
    H. 18
    J. 19
    K. 21

57. On Peter's homework assignment of a state map, $\frac{1}{2}$ inch represents 12 miles. If a distance is 84 miles, how many inches long will it be in Peter's map?
    A. 3
    B. 3.5
    C. 5
    D. 5.5
    E. 6

58. Which of the following numbers has the digit 3 in the hundredths place?
    F. 315
    G. 3.15
    H. 0.0315
    J. 0.00315
    K. 0.000315

59. Approximately what percent of 81 is 36?
    A. 34
    B. 44
    C. 54
    D. 64
    E. 74

60. What is the fifth term in the arithmetic sequence 21, 17, 13, 9…
    F. 5
    G. 6
    H. 7
    J. 8
    K. 9

Reading

Questions 1-10 pertain to the following passage:

<u>The Lesson</u>
    When I was in college I took a Psychology of Film course that was co-taught by a psychology professor, Professor Smith, and a film studies professor, Professor Ruiz. They switched off each week; one week Professor Ruiz would introduce us to a particular film or a genre of films, the next week Professor Smith would talk to us about the way in which that film or genre appealed, or didn't appeal, to audiences and what that says about who we are as a culture and what we get from watching movies. One of the things that Professor Smith touched on regularly as an aspect of movie-watching was the societal cohesion and community building that comes from the shared experience of having watched the same movie. He talked about how we bond by having similar experiences and similar reactions to those experiences.

    One week it was Professor Ruiz' turn to lecture us but Professor Smith told us that she was unable to come to class that day because she was attending a conference. He said he would introduce us to the film that we'd been assigned for that class. We'd all watched it the previous week. It was a movie I had never heard of, made in the early 1970s. I didn't think it was particularly good and from my brief conversations with other students, it didn't seem like anyone else had either. Professor Smith started the lecture in an unusual way. He asked us to write down our name and how we rated the film, from one to ten, ten being the best. I rated it a four. He said he would collect the papers at the end of the class.

    He spent the next hour telling us about the reception the movie had when it came out: he said it was a huge success and got great reviews. He told us that most respected reviewers thought the film was one of the most influential movies ever made and that it challenged and stretched the art form in a way that has yet to be matched. With 30 minutes remaining of the class period, he remembered the papers on which we'd rated the movie. He asked us to pass them in, but said that if any of us, upon reflection, wanted to change our rating, we could do it before passing it in. It seemed like all of us wanted to change our rating. I certainly did; I changed my rating to an 8 after hearing Professor Smith talk about how fabulous people thought the movie was.

    I looked up, ready to pass in my paper and saw Professor Smith smiling at us. He told us he wasn't going to collect our papers. He said that the lesson for that day had been about the power of other people's opinions to influence our own. He noted that he hadn't told us anything substantive about the movie that could have affected our opinion; all that he told us was that well-respected people thought that the movie was extraordinary. We spent the rest of the class talking about whether it's okay to rely on other people's opinions. As he pointed out, it's certainly wise to listen to them and consider the possibility that we've gotten something wrong if many smart people disagree with us. But we also talked about the importance of knowing what you're doing. Being persuaded by the credentials of someone else is very different from being persuaded by the arguments of someone else. Both can be okay but the lesson I took from that class was that, if you want to be a critical thinker, it's necessary to know the difference.

1. Which of the following can reasonably be inferred from the passage?
    A. The movie the author discusses was nominated for an award when it came out.
    B. The movie the author discusses was included in the class to support the lesson about the power of other people's opinions to influence our own, rather than for its artistic merit.
    C. The author became a film reviewer.
    D. The author doesn't believe it is okay to rely on other people's opinions.

2. According to the passage, which of the following is true?
    F. The professors asked the students to rate every movie on a scale of one-to-ten.
    G. The movie discussed in the piece was released in 1979.
    H. The author changed his or her rating of the movie after hearing the professor's lecture.
    J. Both professors were in class the day the author discusses in the passage.

3. Which of the following is most likely the reason for the author's inclusion of the description of the professor's smile?
    A. To show professor has a good sense of humor
    B. To show professor was nice
    C. To show professor liked his students
    D. To suggest things weren't as they seemed

4. Which of the following statements is true regarding the teacher's claim that the movie got great reviews?
    F. It is not necessarily true; it was possibly just said in order to teach the lesson the Professor wanted to convey.
    G. It is necessarily true.
    H. It is necessarily false.
    J. The professor's statement was made up by the author.

5. What does the author say is necessary to know if you want to be a critical thinker?
    A. the difference between truth and lies
    B. the difference between film critics and the general public
    C. the difference between being persuaded by someone's credentials versus by their arguments
    D. the difference between good and bad films

6. Which of the following does the author say Professor Ruiz discussed regularly in class?
    F. the difference between good and bad movies
    G. movies from the 1970s
    H. reviewers
    J. social cohesion and community building through movie watching

7. Which of the following can be inferred from the passage?
    A. the author is a senior in college
    B. the author never went to college
    C. the author is no longer in college
    D. the author looks forward to going to college

8. According to Professor Smith, why didn't Professor Ruiz lecture that day?
    F. It was not her turn.
    G. She was attending a conference.
    H. She didn't like the movie under discussion.
    J. She didn't like the lesson plan.

9. Which word is most nearly synonymous with the meaning of "critical" in the last sentence of the passage?
   A. fault-finding
   B. analytical
   C. disparaging
   D. derogatory

10. According to the author, how many of the students appeared to want to change the rating they'd given the film?
    F. none
    G. ten
    H. less than half
    J. all

Questions 11-20 pertain to the following passage:

Joseph Smith and Mormonism

Joseph Smith, Jr., born in Vermont in 1805, was the founder of Mormonism. In the late 1820s, he claimed to have been visited by an angel named Moroni who led him to a book on golden plates that was buried on a hill near Smith's home. This book recorded the history of God's dealings with indigenous inhabitants of the Americas. Smith claimed to have taken possession of the plates which he said were written in "Reformed Egyptian."

A neighbor of Smith's, Martin Harris, transcribed the translation of the plates as Smith dictated. The resulting 116 manuscripts were lost by Harris. Smith then dictated to his wife his first written revelation which assured Smith that if he repented the loss of the manuscript, God would allow him to redo the translation. The Book of Mormon was finally published in 1830; Martin Harris financed the publication by mortgaging his farm.

In April of 1830, Joseph Smith formally created the Church of Christ. In the early 1830s he also published the Book of Moses and a collection of his earlier revelations published as the Book of Commandments.

In 1832, Smith was twenty-six years old and leading a church of about one thousand members. He faced difficulties internally with the management of such a large organization and with disaffected former followers who accused him of various misdeeds. He also faced opposition to his revelations and religious beliefs externally. That year, he was beaten, tarred and feathered and narrowly escaped being castrated.

Smith courted controversy with his institution of plural marriage. In 1841 he secretly married a second wife, and in less than three years after that may have married about thirty additional women. About a third of those new wives were teenagers. Smith faced opposition to this institution from the outer world, whose fears of Mormonism were felt to be confirmed by this disturbing practice. His wife, Emma Smith, intensely disliked this aspect of her marriage. Emma Smith, in fact, frequently denied that her husband had been a polygamist.

Another opponent of polygamy, William Law, had been one of Smith's greatest supporters. Disagreeing with Smith over plural marriage as well as other issues, Law gave testimony that resulted in three indictments being brought against Smith, including one accusing him of polygamy. Law then published a newspaper called the Nauvoo Expositor that attacked Smith. Smith, then Mayor of the town in which the paper was published, ordered the city marshal to destroy the paper. Smith, facing criminal charges for the destruction of the press, surrendered and went to jail. A mob stormed the jail and Smith was killed.

In the early 21st Century, there may be as many as 14 million members of denominations arising from Joseph Smith's teachings. The Church of Jesus Christ of Latter Day Saints alone claims a membership of thirteen million.

11. According to the passage, how was the publication of the Book of Mormon financed?
    A. God allowed him to redo the translation.
    B. Smith led a church of about 1,000 members.
    C. Martin Harris mortgaged his farm.
    D. Smith dictated the book to Martin Harris.

12. According to the passage, what political office did Smith hold when he ordered the destruction of the newspaper?
    F. City Marshal
    G. Mayor
    H. Expositor
    J. Supreme Leader

13. According to the passage, with what issue did Smith court controversy?
    A. his claim to have been visited by the angel Moroni
    B. his claim that the gold plates were written in "Reformed Egyptian"
    C. his institution of plural marriage
    D. his collection of early writings

14. According to the passage, what did the Book of Mormon describe?
    F. God's dealings with indigenous Americans
    G. the angel Moroni
    H. the language "Reformed Egyptian"
    J. the hill near Smith's home

15. Which of the following is not a text published at the behest of Smith?
    A. Book of Mormon
    B. Book of Moses
    C. Book of Commandments
    D. Book of Moroni

16. According to the passage, how many members does the Church of Jesus Christ of Latter Day Saints say it has?
    F. 116
    G. 1,000
    H. 13,000,000
    J. 14,000,000

17. Which of the following is true according to the passage?
    A. In 1832, Smith was 26 years old.
    B. In 1820, he created the Church of Christ.
    C. In 1840, he had more than 30 wives.
    D. In 1805, he founded Mormonism.

18. According to the passage, which of the following was an opponent of polygamy?
    F. angel Moroni
    G. Martin Harris
    H. Nauvoo Expositor
    J. William Law

19. As of the year 2000, how long had the Church of Christ been in existence?
    A. 270 years
    B. 170 years
    C. 100 years
    D. 70 years

20. According to the passage, which of the following statements is true of Emma Smith?
    F. She never legally became Smith's wife.
    G. She was not Mormon.
    H. She disliked polygamy.
    J. She divorced Smith.

Questions 21-30 pertain to the following passage:

Emily Dickinson

The American poet Emily Dickinson was born in 1830 and lived to the age of 55, passing away before seeing the majority of her work (almost 1,800 poems) published. Less than a dozen of her poems were published in her lifetime.

After Dickinson's death, her younger sister Lavinia discovered the vast store of poems Dickinson had penned. Lavinia was determined to have them published, and the first volume was published in 1890, four years after Dickinson's death. Dickinson has remained continuously in print since then.

Dickinson made extensive use of dashes and unconventional capitalization and she did not write in the traditional iambic pentameter. While some of her contemporary critics found fault in her departure from 19th-century poetic form, modern critics find deliberate aesthetic significance in her unusual style.

In the first publications of Dickinson's works, the poems were heavily edited to make the punctuation and capitalization more conventional. It was not until 1955 that the first scholarly publication was issued, leaving Dickinson's poems almost entirely unchanged from how she had written them in her manuscripts.

Dickinson's poems often employed humor, and the subject matter often concerned flowers, death and dying, the teaching of Jesus Christ, and the mind and spirit (often referred to as the "undiscovered continent").

Emily Dickinson is now a significant figure in American literature and culture. She is widely acknowledged to be a major American poet, standing alongside Walt Whitman, Wallace Stevens, Robert Frost and T.S. Eliot. Her work is taught in American literature and poetry classes in the United States from middle school to college. The Emily Dickinson Museum was created in 2003 when ownership of a family home was transferred to Amherst College.

21. Which of the following was *not* a common subject matter in Dickinson's poems?
    A. her sister
    B. flowers
    C. death
    D. teachings of Jesus Christ

22. According to the passage, which of the following is true of Dickinson's style?
    F. she used commas extensively
    G. she used dashes extensively
    H. she used parentheses extensively
    J. she used colons extensively

23. According to the passage, which of the following is true about Dickinson's place in American literature?
    A. She used to be a significant figure in American literature.
    B. She is now a significant figure in American literature.
    C. She was never a significant figure in American literature.
    D. She will become a significant figure in American literature.

24. How many of Dickinson's poems were published in her lifetime?
    F. none
    G. almost 12
    H. almost 1,800
    J. all of them

25. According to the passage, with what aspect of her work did her contemporary critics find fault?
    A. her humor
    B. her departure from 19th-century poetic form
    C. her obsession with mortality
    D. her young age

26. What did the "undiscovered continent" refer to in Dickinson's poems?
    F. Jesus Christ
    G. poetry
    H. the mind and spirit
    J. love

27. According to the passage, why was her poetry heavily edited at first?
    A. to make her punctuation and capitalization more conventional
    B. to make her punctuation and subject matter more conventional
    C. to make her subject matter and capitalization more conventional
    D. to make her humor and punctuation more conventional

28. In what year was the Emily Dickinson Museum created?
    F. 1830
    G. 1885
    H. 1955
    J. 2003

29. Which of the following is not an American poet named in the passage?
    A. Wallace Stevens
    B. Walt Whitman
    C. Ezra Pound
    D. Robert Frost

30. In what year were Dickinson's poems first published in a form almost unchanged from her manuscripts?
    F. 1830
    G. 1885
    H. 1955
    J. 2003

Questions 31-40 pertain to the following passage:

Comets

Comets are bodies that orbit the sun. They are distinguishable from asteroids by the presence of coma or tails. In the outer solar system, comets remain frozen and are so small that they are difficult to detect from Earth. As a comet approaches the inner solar system, solar radiation causes the materials within the comet to vaporize and trail off the nuclei. The released dust and gas forms a fuzzy atmosphere called the coma, and the force exerted on the coma causes a tail to form, pointing away from the sun.

Comet nuclei are made of ice, dust, rock and frozen gases and vary widely in size: from 100 meters or so to tens of kilometers across. The comas may be even larger than the Sun. Because of their low mass, they do not become spherical and have irregular shapes.

There are over 3,500 known comets, and the number is steadily increasing. This represents only a small portion of the total comets existing, however. Most comets are too faint to be visible without the aid of a telescope; the number of comets visible to the naked eye is around one a year.

Comets leave a trail of solid debris behind them. If a comet's path crosses the Earth's path, there will likely be meteor showers as Earth passes through the trail of debris.

Many comets and asteroids have collided into Earth. Some scientists believe that comets hitting Earth about 4 billion years ago brought a significant proportion of the water in Earth's oceans. There are still many near-Earth comets.

Most comets have oval shaped orbits that take them close to the Sun for part of their orbit and then out further into the Solar System for the remainder of the orbit. Comets are often classified according to the length of their orbital period: short period comets have orbital periods of less than 200 years, long period comets have orbital periods of more than 200 years, single apparition comets have trajectories which cause them to permanently leave the solar system after passing the Sun once.

31. What does the passage *not* list as a component of comet nuclei?
    A. solar radiation
    B. dust
    C. frozen gases
    D. rock

32. According to the passage, what do some scientists believe brought a significant proportion of the water in the Earth's oceans?
    F. Comets' released gas and dust
    G. Comets exiting in the solar system
    H. Comet collisions with the Sun
    J. Comet collisions with Earth

33. What does the passage claim distinguishes comets from asteroids?
    A. The make-up of their nuclei
    B. The presence of coma or tails
    C. Their orbital periods
    D. Their irregular shapes

34. What would a comet with an orbital period of 1,000 years be called?
    F. a short period comet
    G. a long period comet
    H. a single apparition comet
    J. an elliptical comet

35. According to the passage, which of the following is true?
    A. There are 350 known comets and the number is steadily increasing.
    B. There are 3,500 known comets and the number is staying the same.
    C. There are 3,500 known comets and many more comets that aren't known.
    D. Most comets are visible to the naked eye.

36. According to the passage, what makes up the coma?
    F. released dust and gas
    G. a meteor shower
    H. asteroids
    J. rock

37. According to the passage, why do comets have irregular shapes?
    A. because they are not spherical
    B. because they have orbital periods
    C. because of their low mass
    D. because of their tails

38. What does the passage claim about the size of comets?
    F. Some are tens of kilometers across and the coma can be larger than the Sun
    G. Some are tens of kilometers across and the coma is never larger than the Sun
    H. Some are 100 meters across and the coma is never larger than the Sun
    J. The smallest comet is at least a kilometer and the coma can be larger than the Sun

39. According to the passage, what shape is the orbit of most comets?
    A. circular
    B. square
    C. linear
    D. oval

40. According to the passage, why are comets in the outer solar system difficult to detect from Earth?
    F. They are not in orbit.
    G. They are frozen.
    H. They have irregular shapes.
    J. They are small.

Science

Questions 1-5 pertain to the following information:

Students on the cross-country Team at Little Star High School tracked the results of three different training programs. The team of 18 students split into 3 equal-sized groups and spent 5 weeks training apart. Each group was responsible for maintaining a chart of weekly runs with speed and distances noted.

Group 1 followed training Program A and had time results (in minutes) as follows:

Student	Run 1 5 mile	Run 2 7 mile	Run 3 5 mile	Run 4 10 mile	Run 5 15 mile
1	30	44	29	70	99
2	31	48	30	70	100
3	25	42	24	59	83
4	27	46	26	64	88
5	35	51	34	81	115
6	29	41	28	68	96

Group 2 followed training Program B and had results as follows:

Student	Run 1 10 mile	Run 2 3 mile	Run 3 10 mile	Run 4 3 mile	Run 5 15 mile
1	73	18	73	18	103
2	74	19	74	18	107
3	62	23	62	21	88
4	67	21	67	20	94
5	84	27	81	29	120
6	72	19	72	24	99

Group 3 followed training Program C and had results as follows:

Student	Run 1 3 mile	Run 2 6 mile	Run 3 9 mile	Run 4 12 mile	Run 5 15 mile
1	18	41	59	105	121
2	19	43	62	107	115
3	23	46	69	115	120
4	21	43	64	107	108
5	27	53	80	133	115
6	19	39	58	97	100

1. In which of the training programs did a student run 5 miles in 24 minutes?
    A. Program A
    B. Program B
    C. Program C
    D. none of the programs

2. In which of the training programs did Student 1 twice run 3 miles in 18 minutes?
    F. Program A
    G. Program B
    H. Program C
    J. none of the programs

3. In which of the training programs did a student run 10 miles in 59 minutes?
   A. Program A
   B. Program B
   C. Program C
   D. none of the programs

4. In which of the training programs did Student 4 take 109 minutes to complete a run?
   F. Program A
   G. Program B
   H. Program C
   J. none of the programs

5. If the goal of the training program is to enable people to run 15 miles as fast as possible, in which order are the programs the best?
   A. Program A, then C, then B
   B. Program A, then B, then C
   C. Program B, then A, then C
   D. Program B, then C, then A

Questions 6-12 pertain to the following information:

Scientists disagree about the benefits of adaptations of many different animals. Two scientists discuss one adaptation of the fish of the coral-reef.

Scientist 1
   The brilliant displays of colors of the fish of the coral-reef: scarlet, rose, yellow, turquoise, emerald and dozens of others, serve as camouflage for the fish living in the color complexity of the reef. We are incorrect if we analyze fish coloration by human eye standards; things look very different from the fishes' point of view. Fish cannot discern the yellow/ green color family with the particularity that the human eye can so, for example, a yellow trumpet fish nearly matches the green of the average coral reef. And the blue of the blue-and-yellow angel fish matches the bluish backgrounds a fish sees when looking to the distance in deep water. We need to understand the camouflage effect by how the fish see the world.

Scientist 2
   In fish, as with many other animal species (peacocks, butterflies, snakes, etc...), the brilliant colors of the body are there to be seen and paid attention to. The bright colors might send flaunting messages: come-ons to potential mates or warnings to possible predators that the fish has distasteful or toxic flesh. It has also been suggested that the bright and varied colors might act as a kind of ecosystem color-coding that lets all the fish species that share a reef keep track of who is who.

6. Which of the following phrases best describe the major point of difference between the two scientists' viewpoints?
   F. adaptations in many different animals
   G. the function of coloration in coral-reef fish.
   H. the fish of the coral-reef
   J. the different colors of coral-reef fish

7. According to Scientist 1,
    A. fish don't care about color differences
    B. fish aren't threatened by color differences
    C. fish perceive color differently than humans
    D. fish aren't attracted to color differences

8. Which of the following is the best synonym for the word "flaunting" as used in the passage?
    F. showy
    G. modest
    H. camouflaged
    J. discreet

9. With what other animal does Scientist 2 not compare fish?
    A. snakes
    B. butterflies
    C. beetles
    D. peacocks

10. According to Scientist 1, which color family can fish not discriminate as well as humans can?
    F. blue/ green
    G. yellow/ green
    H. yellow/ blue
    J. scarlet/ rose

11. According to Scientist 2, which of the following is true?
    A. The bright colors might send predators the message that the fish are ferocious.
    B. The bright colors might send predators the message that the fish are toxic.
    C. The bright colors might send predators the message that the fish are camouflaged.
    D. The bright colors might send predators the message that the fish are fast.

12. Which of the following is true?
    F. Scientist 1 suggests that fish coloration may be a kind of ecosystem color-coding.
    G. Scientist 2 suggests that fish coloration may be a kind of ecosystem color-coding.
    H. Scientist 1 suggests that the fish are actually all the same color.
    J. Scientist 2 suggests that the fish are actually all the same color.

Questions 13-17 pertain to the following information:

A scientist studies the effect of a placebo on public speaking performance. A group of 20 self-professed nervous public speakers all give an initial 5-minute talk to the other participants. Then, half the group is given a pill that they are told will make them more comfortable with public speaking while the other half is given nothing. The participants give another 5-minute talk. Both talks are rated by the other participants in the group on a scale of 1-5, 5 being the best and this rating is averaged. The results are as follows:

	Participant	1st Talk	2nd Talk
Placebo Group	1	3	3
	2	2	4
	3	1	3
	4	1	2
	5	3	3
	6	2	2
	7	4	3
	8	3	3
	9	2	3
	10	2	2
No-treatment Group	11	1	2
	12	2	2
	13	3	3
	14	3	3
	15	2	3
	16	4	3
	17	3	2
	18	2	3
	19	2	2
	20	4	3

13. How many of the participants in the Placebo Group improved their rating from the 1st talk to the 2nd talk?

   A. 1
   B. 2
   C. 3
   D. 4

14. How many participants in the non-Placebo Group improved their rating from the 1st talk to the 2nd talk?

   F. 1
   G. 2
   H. 3
   J. 4

15. How many of the participants in the Placebo Group received a lower rating from the 1st talk to the 2nd talk?

   A. 1
   B. 2
   C. 3
   D. 4

16. How many of the participants in the non-Placebo Group received a lower rating from the 1st talk to the 2nd talk?
    F. 1
    G. 2
    H. 3
    J. 4

17. Which of the following participants received the most points in his or her combined two talks?
    A. Participant 1
    B. Participant 2
    C. Participant 7
    D. Participant 8

Questions 18-22 pertain to the following information:

A scientist at a zoo studies the impact of number of close relationships on longevity of baboons. She studies a group of 13 baboons and counts a close relationship as any proximal contact with a duration of 15 minutes or more, more than 3 times a week for 3 consecutive weeks. The contact must be positive, I.E., it does not count as contact if is predominantly based in aggression.

She records the age of the baboons at death. Her results can be summarized as follows:

Baboon	Number of Close Relationships	Age at time of death (in years)
1	5	Living
2	7	13
3	5	Living
4	4	3
5	9	18
6	6	12
7	5	living
8	4	living
9	5	12
10	7	16
11	10	living
12	6	living
13	6	13

18. What is the average age at time of death for the baboons with 7 close relationships?
    F. 13
    G. 14.5
    H. 15.5
    J. 16

19. How many close relationships did the longest living baboon have?
    A. 8
    B. 9
    C. 10
    D. 11

20. How many close relationships did the youngest deceased baboon have?
    F. 3
    G. 4
    H. 5
    J. 6

21. How many close relationships did the baboon that lived to be 16 have?
    A. 5
    B. 6
    C. 7
    D. 8

22. Which living baboon has the most close relationships?
    F. Baboon 1
    G. Baboon 3
    H. Baboon 9
    J. Baboon 11

Questions 23-28 pertain to the following passage:

Bats are one of the largest and most diverse mammal orders – accounting for one-fifth of all living mammal species. A long-standing question about bats had been about how they evolved. Specifically, scientists have wondered which came first for bats: flight or their sonar system which they use to navigate and hunt for prey. Or, some scientists questioned, did those two attributes evolve together? In 2003, a bat fossil was found that answered that question.

A well-preserved fossil of the most primitive bat species currently known was found in Wyoming in 2003. Dating the rock formation in which the fossil was found put its age at 52 million years. The fossil had a number of surprising characteristics. More claws than modern bats and different limb proportions from those found on bats today suggest that these early bats may have been skilled climbers. But its long fingers, keeled breastbone and other features indicate that it could fly under its own power like bats of today, though probably not as far or as fast.

On the other hand, the bat's skull lacked features in and around the ear that are found in bats that use echolocation. Without echolocation, the bat species most likely used visual, olfactory and audio cues to hunt. Thus the question was resolved: bats could fly before they had sonar.

23. Which is *not* a possible answer to the long-standing question described in this passage?
    A. echolocation evolved first
    B. the ability to fly evolved first
    C. echolocation and the ability to fly evolved simultaneously
    D. neither echolocation nor the ability to fly evolved

24. Which features did the scientists find that suggest that the bat could have flown?
    F. long fingers and keeled breastbone
    G. keeled breastbone and many claws
    H. many claws and long fingers
    J. unusual limb proportions and many claws

25. What features were absent that suggest the bat could not echolocate?
    A. long limbs
    B. features in and around the ear that bats use for echolocation
    C. multiple fingers
    D. keeled breastbone

26. What is the closest meaning for the word "olfactory" as used in the passage?
    F. of or relating to the sense of sight
    G. of or relating to the sense of hearing
    H. of or relating to the sense of sonar
    J. of or relating to the sense of smell

27. How did the scientists estimate the fossil's age?
    A. by comparing it to modern day bat skeletons
    B. by echolocation
    C. by dating the rock formation in which fossil was found
    D. by archaeology

28. Which of the following characteristics suggest that this species of bats were skilled climbers?
    F. long fingers
    G. keeled breastbone
    H. more claws that found on modern bats
    J. less claws than found on modern bats

Questions 29-34 pertain to the following passage:

Two recent studies have indicated that caffeine may reduce beta amyloid, a protein that is a sign of Alzheimer's disease when found in sticky clumps.

The studies followed 55 mice which showed signs of memory loss at an age equivalent to 70 years in a human. Half of the mice received no caffeine; the other half received the mouse equivalent of 5 8-ounce cups of coffee. The half of the mice that received the coffee recovered from their memory loss and had memories the equivalent of mice without dementia.

The findings suggest that caffeine could be more than just a protective strategy to avoid Alzheimer's, but also a treatment for those with the disease. Caffeine also has a number of benefits as treatment: it is generally safe for most people, enters the brain easily and appears to affect the disease directly. Human trials are expected to start soon and are needed to decide whether or not caffeine has a similar effect on people as it does on mice.

29. According to the passage, what might caffeine work to reduce?
    A. treatment
    B. age
    C. beta amyloid
    D. memory

30. The mice received the human equivalent of how many ounces of coffee?
    F. 20
    G. 30
    H. 40
    J. 50

31. According to the passage, which of the following is *not* a benefit of caffeine as treatment?
    A. it enters the blood stream easily
    B. it is generally safe for most people
    C. it appears to affect the disease directly
    D. it enters the brain directly

32. What percentage of the mice in the studies received no caffeine?
    F. 25%
    G. 75%
    H. 50%
    J. 100%

33. According to the passage, which of the following is true?
    A. Beta amyloid is not a protein.
    B. Beta amyloid is not found in sticky clumps.
    C. Beta amyloid is a protein.
    D. Alzheimer's is found in sticky clumps.

34. What was the human age equivalent of the age of the mice studied in the test?
    F. 5
    G. 55
    H. 70
    J. 8

Questions 35-40 pertain the following passage:

   A group of scientists have built a knee-mounted device that can harvest energy from a person's walking power. In the future, the technology should be able to power portable devices such as iPods, GPS locators or mobile phones. In the very near future the technology could help power medical devices such as prosthetic limbs, or implants such as pacemakers. The technology also could someday provide extra energy for military personnel without the added weight of a backpack battery.

   The device, which weighs about 1.6 kilograms, can generate an average of five watts of electricity with minimal extra effort on the part of the walker. It gets its energy not from the power used to move the leg forward, but from the energy put into slowing down the knee at the end of a person's step. The concept is similar to that used by hybrid-electric cars which recycle power from braking.

   Tests of the device have shown that it requires little extra metabolic power to produce energy. Energy is required to carry the bulky device itself though, so scientists developing the product are working on making it smaller and more lightweight.

35. According to the passage, which of the following is true?
    A. The device weighs about 1.6 kilograms and requires a great deal of extra metabolic power to produce energy.
    B. The device weighs about 1.6 pounds and requires a great deal of extra metabolic power to produce energy.
    C. the device weighs about 1.6 kilograms and requires little extra metabolic power to produce energy.
    D. The device weighs about 1.6 pounds and requires little extra metabolic power to produce energy.

36. According to the passage, from where does the device get its energy?
    F. the power to move the leg forward
    G. energy put into slowing down the knee
    H. a backpack battery
    J. a pacemaker

37. According to the passage, how many watts of electricity can the device generate on average?
    A. 3
    B. 4
    C. 5
    D. 6

38. Which of the following is not listed as something the technology could help power?
    F. iPod
    G. pacemaker
    H. backpack battery
    J. prosthetic limb

39. What improvements are scientists working on?
    A. making it fit in a backpack
    B. making it generate more electricity
    C. giving it extra metabolic power
    D. making it smaller and more lightweight

40. To what other technology does the author compare the device described in the passage?
    F. hybrid-electric cars
    G. pacemakers
    H. GPS locators
    J. backpack battery

Answer Key and Explanations

English

Number	Answer	Number	Answer	Number	Answer
1	C	26	H	51	C
2	G	27	C	52	H
3	D	28	J	53	A
4	J	29	A	54	G
5	A	30	G	55	C
6	G	31	D	56	G
7	A	32	G	57	C
8	F	33	A	58	G
9	B	34	H	59	B
10	H	35	C	60	F
11	B	36	J	61	B
12	J	37	A	62	G
13	B	38	G	63	A
14	G	39	B	64	F
15	D	40	J	65	D
16	G	41	B	66	G
17	D	42	F	67	D
18	F	43	D	68	F
19	C	44	G	69	D
20	G	45	A	70	F
21	B	46	H	71	C
22	J	47	D	72	G
23	A	48	G	73	D
24	J	49	A	74	H
25	B	50	J	75	A

1. C: The restoration of the frescoes happened in the past (the 10th century), so the sentence verb should be in the past tense.

2. G: *The chapel* is singular so the possessive form should have the apostrophe before the *s*.

3. D: The subject of this sentence, *the most recent restoration*, is singular so the verb needs to be singular as well.

4. J: The forms of the verbs need to be parallel.

5. A: This sentence is correct as written.

6. G: This sentence needs the past tense of the verb *to include*.

7. A: This sentence is correct as written.

8. F: This sentence is correct as written.

9. B: It is correct to say *in addition*, or to say *additionally*, but *in additionally* is not a proper construction.

10. H: A list of adjectives modifying the same noun should be separated by commas, not a hyphen.

11. B: The action described in the sentence happened in the past so the verb needs to be in the past tense.

12. J: The action described in the sentence happened in the past so the verb needs to be in the past tense.

13. B: *As a result* is the correct form of this expression.

14. G: *Michelangelo* is singular so the possessive form should have the apostrophe before the *s*.

15. D: An adjective is needed to modify *the assumption*. The word *broad* is an adjective and is correct where *broadly*, an adverb, is not.

16. G: *On the market* is the correct version of the colloquial expression.

17. D: The sentence needs an adverb to modify the verb *follow*.

18. F: No change is needed. The infinitive form is correct.

19. C: The word needed in the sentence is the contraction of *it is*, which is correctly written as *it's*.

20. G: The meaning of the sentence indicates that the correct word is *though*.

21. B: The form of the word *easy* needed in this sentence is an adjective, *easy*, not an adverb, *easily*.

22. J: *Want* is the verb tense that agrees with the subject *we*.

23. A: *In the meantime* is the correct phrase.

24. J: This sentence needs the infinitive form of the verb *implement*.

25. B: The correct form of the verb in this sentence is *reduce*.

26. H: The subject of the sentence is *Lemon*; the correct form of the verb that agrees with the subject is *acts*.

27. C: The plural *these* correctly modifies the plural *things*.

28. J: The sentence uses the expression *fun of…*.

29. A: No change is needed. *Our* is the correct word choice.

30. G: The singular *step* is the correct word choice for this sentence.

31. D: *Are estimated* is the correct verb construction for this sentence.

32. G: The word *each* indicates that *year* should be singular.

33. A: The sentence is correct as written.

34. H: The word *A* indicates that *number* should be singular.

35. C: The verb tense should be in the present.

36. J: *Hours* should be in the plural.

37. A: The sentence is correct as written.

38. G: The correct expression is *even more than*.

39. B: The phrase *in the past* should be set off by a comma.

40. J: This sentence describes an action in the past and thus needs a verb in past tense.

41. B: This sentence describes an action in the past and thus needs a verb in past tense.

42. F: The sentence is correct as written.

43. D: The correct form of the comparative adjective is *more comfortable*.

44. G: One explains something *to* another person, not *on, in,* or *at* them.

45. A: The sentence is correct as written.

46. H: The word choice needs to modify *famous*; *internationally* is the only option that does so.

47. D: The colloquial expression is *life on a ship*.

48. G: The parenthetical should be set off by commas on both sides.

49. A: The sentence is correct as written.

50. J: The phrase needs to describe when Josephine accepts her father's wishes; *at first* does this.

51. C: This is the correct spelling for the word that describes having an auditory experience of something.

52. H: This sentence needs the infinitive form of the verb *to declare*.

53. A: The sentence is correct as written.

54. G: This sentence describes an action in the past and thus needs a verb in past tense.

55. C: The expression sought in the sentence is one that indicates that something is not the case anymore. *No longer* is that expression.

56. G: The correct word in this sentence is a singular possessive.

57. C: This sentence describes an action in the past and thus needs a verb in past tense.

58. G: *Favorable* is the correct word choice as an adjective to describe a positive review.

59. B: The verb of the sentence needs to be in the present tense.

60. F: The sentence is correct as written.

61. B: Parenthetical comments need to be set off by matching punctuation marks. In this case, a dash was used at the end and needs to be used at the beginning as well.

62. G: No comparison is made in the sentence so it doesn't make sense to use a comparative adjective.

63. A: The sentence is correct as written.

64. F: The sentence is correct as written.

65. D: The sentence requires a singular noun. *D* is the only choice that uses one.

66. G: In the passage as written, the first sentence in the fourth paragraph describes *Another* advantage. This paragraph would be more clear if the other advantage described (meeting the high need for city housing) came first.

67. D: The sixth paragraph discusses the shotgun home's role in the idea of Southern life, so the subject matter fits. Also, the sixth paragraph is the concluding paragraph and this sentence works as a concluding sentence.

68. F: The sentence is correct as written.

69. D: The verb in this sentence needs to be in the past tense.

70. F: The sentence is correct as written.

71. C: The verb in this sentence needs to be in the past tense.

72. G: Answer *G* provides the necessary subject verb agreement of *neighborhoods...contain*.

73. D: When listing more than two nouns, the correct way to refer to them is *all* rather than *each*.

74. H: The verb in this sentence needs to be in the past tense.

75. A: The sentence is correct as written.

Mathematics

Number	Answer	Number	Answer	Number	Answer
1	C	21	C	41	D
2	F	22	H	42	H
3	D	23	C	43	A
4	G	24	H	44	G
5	A	25	A	45	B
6	H	26	J	46	H
7	D	27	C	47	B
8	F	28	G	48	F
9	B	29	D	49	C
10	H	30	F	50	J
11	A	31	D	51	B
12	G	32	J	52	H
13	B	33	C	53	B
14	J	34	F	54	J
15	A	35	D	55	A
16	F	36	G	56	H
17	D	37	B	57	B
18	H	38	J	58	H
19	A	39	B	59	B
20	H	40	J	60	F

1. C: For the trim to cover the entire perimeter of the quilt it would need to be 7 + 6 + 7 + 6 = 26 feet long.

2. F: 74 x 5 = 370. 76 + 80 + 69 + 71 = 296. 370 – 296 = 74.

3. D: 1 2/3 + 2 3/7 = 5/3 + 17/7 = 35/21 + 51/21 = 86/21 = 4 2/21

4. G: If 3x – 2 = 5x – 14, then 2x = 12 so x = 6

5. A: 8% of $64,000 = 8/100 x 64,000 = 5,120. Mathilda will be making $64,000 + $5120, or $69,120. This is closest to $69,000.

6. H: If Mary biked three times as much as David, she biked 30 miles. She biked it in $\frac{1}{2}$ of the time David biked in, or 2 hours. 30 miles in 2 hours is a rate of 15 mph.

7. D: Remember to multiply out these equations using the order FOIL (first, outside, inside, last). Using this approach, we get 4x2+ 8x – 3x – 6 or 4x2 + 5x – 6

8. F: The absolute value of -4 squared is 16. The absolute value of -7 is 7. Therefore solve for the equation 16 + 7 – 2. The answer is 21.

9. B: If a distance of 45 feet wide is split into two portions, one twice as long as the other, we can write this mathematically as 2x + x = 45 or 3x = 45. x (the width of the smaller room) then = 15.

10. H: If Abe goes 3 miles in one hour, he goes half of that or $1\frac{1}{2}$ miles in one half hour. Similarly, Beatriz can go 2 miles in one half hour. The answer therefore = $2 - 1\frac{1}{2} = \frac{1}{2}$.

11. A: x – 2 + x – 1 + x + x + 1 + x + 2 = 5x = 390. x = 38

12. G: 30xy is not a multiple of 4x. The next smallest figure listed is 60xy which is a multiple of all the numbers given and is therefore the correct answer.

13. B: The absolute value of 8 – 7 is 1. The absolute value of 7 – 8 is also 1. 1 – 1 = 0

14. J: Robert paid $9 in drop-off fees. If he paid $130 total and we use x to represent the number of hours of childcare he paid for, that means that 130 = 9 + 11x. 121 = 11x. x = 11.

15. A: -2 squared is 4. 4(-4) + 2(8) = -16 + 16 = 0

16. F: Note that Anna's route creates a right triangle. Use the Pythagorean Theorem to calculate the answer. 82 + 62 = x2. 64 + 36 = x2. 100 = x2. x = 10.

17. D: 7 + 7 + z = 27. z = 27 – 14. z = 13.

18. H: Allison spends $200 a month on gas. That $200 is 80% of her transportation costs. 200 = 80/100 x. x = 250. 250 is 1/10 of her salary, so her monthly salary is $2,500. The monthly salary x 12 equals her annual salary of $30,000.

19. A: One hour and 39 minutes equals 99 minutes. 99 divided by 33 is 3.

20. H: We know x has to be a negative number because if it's not, the answer for the equation would be zero rather than 14. If x is negative, what number plus itself equals 14. This can be written 2x = 14. Therefore, x = -7.

21. C: 65% of applicants historically passed the written portion of the application. 65% of 100 is 65. 40% of those 65 passed the oral portion. 40% of 65 = 40/100 x 65 = 26.

22. H: 18.00 + 18.50 + 19.99 + 15.39 = 71.88. 71.88/ 4 = 17.97

23. C: $19.99 - $15.39 = $4.60

24. H: If $\frac{3}{4}$x = 5.25, then x = 7.00. 5/3 x 7.00 = approximately 11.66

25. A: The number of people surveyed is 33 + 64 + 13 = 110. 33/110 = 3/10

26. J: 17 feet and 8 inches = (17 x 12) + 8 = 212 inches. 212/2 = 106 inches. Expressed in feet, that means each half is 8 feet, 10 inches.

27. C: (9/5 x 20) + 32 = 36 + 32 = 68

28. G: 2W + 2(W + 14) = 92. 2W + 2W + 28 = 92. 4W = 64. W = 16

29. D: (78 + 95 + x)/3 has to be at least equal to 90. Solving for that, (78 + 95 + x) = 270. 173 + x = 270. x = 97

30. F: The debt has changed by $13 plus $8 = $21

31. D: 15% of $49.95 = 15/100 x 49.95 = $7.4925, or approximately $7.50

32. J: 6 cubed is 6 x 6 x 6 = 216

33. C: The number of students who chose either turkey or egg salad is 45 + 15 = 60. 60/180 = 1/3, or approximately 33%.

34. F: 60/180 = x/420. 1/3 = x/420. 3x = 420. x = 140

35. D: The ratio indicates the number of people who chose veggie (60) to the number of people who chose turkey (45). 60:45 = 4:3

36. G: Think of the perfect squares closest to the square root of 71. The square root of 64 is 8; the square root of 81 is 9. 81 is larger than 71 so the answer must be 8.

37. B: Sarah used up 8 stickers by putting one on each page. She has 8 stickers remaining. Since every page now needs three stickers to be complete, divide 3 into 8 to see how many pages she can fill. 3 goes into 8 twice with a remainder of 2, so she can fill two pages completely full of stickers.

38. J: The club earned a total of 61 x $10 = $610 through the sale of play tickets. Of that, each child received $610/10 = $61. Since each child needed to come up with a total of $525, the answer is $525 - $61, or $464.

39. B: To get the correct answer, make sure to count the decimal points.

40. J: Charlie received a total of $13.75, of which $10 was his base allowance, leaving $3.75 as pay for doing additional chores. $3.75 divided by $0.75, the amount he gets for doing each chore, is 5.

41. D: $14 - x = 73$ is the same as $x = 14 - 73 = -59$

42. H: Sophie needs to cover an area of 8 x 15 = 120 square feet. Four gallons covers 36 x 4 = 144 square feet. She needs four gallons because the next lesser amount, 3 gallons, only covers 108 square feet.

43. A: 18% of 36,000 is 6,480. One half of that is 3,240.

44. G: $3x - 2 = 5x - 12$ can be written as $2x = 10$ which is the same as $x = 5$.

45. B: $2x + x(x + x + x + x) - x = 2x + x^2 + x^2 + x^2 + x^2 - x$ which = $2x + 4x^2 - x$, which equals $4x^2 + x$

46. H: For questions 46 and 47, note that the only real relevant information given is that Trina lives on Elm Street and that Clara does not live on Elm Street (since she doesn't have a lawn). Thus the statement Clara lives on Elm Street must be false.

47. B: For questions 46 and 47, note that the only real relevant information given is that Trina lives on Elm Street and that Clara does not live on Elm Street (since she doesn't have a lawn). Thus the statement Clara and Trina are not next door neighbors must be true.

48. F: Plug $y = 4$ into $y^2 - 2y - x = 0$, and get $16 - 8 - x = 0$. Or $8 - x = 0$. Thus $x = 8$.

49. C: If we call the membership after it tripled x, and before it tripled y, we know that x = 3y. We also know that x/2 = 75. This means that x = 150. Plugging that into the first equation, we find that y = 50.

50. J: To get a square area enclosed by 40 feet of rope, each side will be $\frac{1}{4}$ of 40 feet, or 10 feet in length. The area enclosed by the sides will then be 10 x 10, or 100, square feet.

51. B: The absolute value of 7 − 4 = 3. The absolute value of 1 − 7 = 6. 3 − 6 = -3.

52. H: If we represent sandwiches by x and drinks by y, we know that 2x + 6y = 8 and 3x + y = 8, or y = 8 - 3x. Solving the first equation for x, we can say that 2x + 6(8 − 3x) = 8. Thus 2x + 48 − 18x = 8, and 16x = 40. Thus x = $2.50

53. B: 8 divided by 3 is 2, with 2 remaining.

54. J: 30/100x = 14,000. Thus x = 20,000

55. A: The absolute value of 7 − 13 is the absolute value of -6, which is 6.

56. H: If the average of the 5 numbers is 9, then (x− 2 + x − 1 + x + x + 1 + x + 2)/5 = 9. This can be written as 5x/5 = 9, or x = 9. If x = 9, the least number in the series is 9 − 2 or 7, and the greatest is x + 2, or 11. 7 + 11 = 18.

57. B: If a distance of 12 miles is represented by a half inch, a distance of 84 miles would be represented by 7 half inches since 84/12 = 7. 7 half inches = 3.5 inches.

58. H: Remember that starting at the decimal point and going right, the place values are tenths, hundredths, thousandths and so on. Thus the decimal 0.0315 has the three in the hundredths place.

59. B: 36/81 = x/100. 81x = 3600. x = approximately 44

60. F: Each number in the list is 4 less than the number that precedes it, which means that 5 appropriately follows 9.

Reading

Number	Answer	Number	Answer
1	B	21	A
2	H	22	G
3	D	23	B
4	F	24	G
5	C	25	B
6	J	26	H
7	C	27	A
8	G	28	J
9	B	29	C
10	J	30	H
11	C	31	A
12	G	32	J
13	C	33	B
14	F	34	G
15	D	35	C
16	H	36	F
17	A	37	C
18	J	38	F
19	B	39	D
20	H	40	J

1. B: The narrator notes that the lesson of the day was about the power of other people's opinions to influence our own. It is clear the movie was included for this purpose.

2. H: The narrator specifically says that he changed his rating of the movie after hearing the professor's lecture.

3. D: The narrator most likely included the description of the smile to suggest that things were not as they seemed to the students, and that the teacher had awareness of this.

4. F: It is clear from the text that the accuracy of the claim that the movie got great reviews was not the subject of the class; the subject of the class that day was the effect of such claims on people who hear them. To give this lesson, the claim doesn't need to be true; it just needs to be believed.

5. C: In the last sentence of the passage the narrator notes that to be a critical thinker it is necessary to know the difference between another person's credentials and another person's arguments.

6. J: In the first paragraph the narrator talks about the social cohesion and community building that can come from watching the same movie.

7. C: The very beginning of the first sentence reads, "When I was in college..." From this we can infer that the narrator attended college and is no longer there.

8. G: The second paragraph of the passage notes that Professor Smith told the class that Professor Ruiz was unable to be there because she was attending a conference.

9. B: Critical here means analytical, judicious, or thoughtful. It does not mean critical in the sense of the other words: disapproving or judgmental.

10. J: In the third paragraph the narrator notes that, "It seemed like all of us wanted to change our rating."

11. C: The last sentence in the second paragraph notes that the publication was financed through the mortgaging of Harris' farm.

12. G: The sixth paragraph notes that Smith was Mayor when he ordered destruction of the press.

13. C: The fifth paragraph notes that Smith courted controversy regarding the issue of plural marriage.

14. F: The first paragraph notes that the Book recorded God's dealings with indigenous Americans.

15. D: Options A, B and C are all texts published at the behest of Smith; the Book of Moroni is not such a text.

16. H: The last sentence of the passage notes that the Church of Jesus Christ Latter Day Saints claims membership of thirteen million.

17. A: The fourth paragraph notes that in 1832, Smith was 26.

18. J: The sixth paragraph names William Law as an opponent of polygamy.

19. B: If the church came into existence in 1830, as of 2000 it would have been in existence 170 years.

20. H: The fifth paragraph describes how Emma Smith disliked polygamy.

21. A: The fifth paragraph lists frequent subject matter of her poems as: flowers, death and dying, the teaching of Jesus Christ and the mind and the spirit.

22. G: The third paragraph notes that she made extensive use of dashes.

23. B: The last paragraph notes that she is now a significant figure in American literature.

24. G: The first paragraph notes that less than 12 of the poems were published in her lifetime.

25. B: Paragraph 3 notes that she was criticized by her contemporaries for departing from 19th Century poetic form.

26. H: Paragraph 5 notes that the mind and spirit were often referred to as the undiscovered continent.

27. A: Paragraph 4 notes that her punctuation and capitalization were edited to be more conventional.

28. J: The last sentence states that the Museum was created in 2003.

29. C: Ezra Pound was not mentioned in the passage.

30. H: Paragraph 4 notes that 1955 was when her poems were first published almost unchanged from her manuscripts.

31. A: Solar radiation is not listed as a component of comet nuclei.

32. J: The passage's 5th paragraph notes that some scientists believe that comet collisions with Earth brought a large proportion of Earth's water.

33. B: The second sentence in the passage notes that comets are distinguishable from asteroids by the presence of comas or tails.

34. G: A comet with an orbit of longer than 200 years is a long period comet.

35. C: The third paragraph notes that there are over 3,500 known comets. It also notes that this represents only a small portion of those in existence.

36. F: The first paragraph explains that a coma is made up of released dust and gas.

37. C: The second paragraph notes that because they have low mass, they don't become spherical and have irregular shapes.

38. F: The second paragraph notes that some comets may be tens of kilometers across. It also notes that comas may be larger than the sun.

39. D: The sixth paragraph notes that most comets have oval shaped orbits.

40. J: The first paragraph notes that comets in the outer solar system are difficult to see because they are small.

Science

Number	Answer	Number	Answer
1	A	21	C
2	G	22	J
3	A	23	D
4	J	24	F
5	B	25	B
6	G	26	J
7	C	27	C
8	F	28	H
9	C	29	C
10	G	30	H
11	B	31	A
12	G	32	H
13	D	33	C
14	H	34	H
15	A	35	C
16	H	36	G
17	C	37	C
18	G	38	H
19	B	39	D
20	G	40	F

1. A: In Run 3 of Program A, Student 3 ran 5 miles in 24 minutes.

2. G: In Runs 2 and 4 of Program B, Student 1 ran 3 miles in 18 minutes.

3. A: In Run 4 of Program A, Student 3 ran 10 miles in 59 minutes.

4. J: Student 4 did not complete a run in 109 minutes in any program.

5. B: Program A yielded the fastest times for 15 mile runs, followed by Program B, then Program C.

6. G: The function of the coloration of the fish is the point of difference between the two scientists.

7. C: According to Scientist 1, fish perceive color differently than humans do.

8. F: Showy is the best synonym for flaunting as used in the passage.

9. C: Scientist 2 does not compare fish to beetles.

10. G: Scientist 1 claims that fish cannot discriminate yellow/green as well as humans can.

11. B: Scientist 2 claims that bright colors might send the warning to predators that a fish's flesh is toxic.

12. G: Scientist 2 suggests that fish coloration may be a kind of ecosystem color-coding.

13. D: Four participants in the Placebo Group improved in the rating given to them (participants 2, 3, 4, and 9).

14. H: Three participants in the non-Placebo Group improved in the rating given to them (participants 11, 15, and 18).

15. A: One participant in the Placebo Group received a lower rating (participant 7).

16. H: Three participants in the non-Placebo Group received a lower rating (participants 16, 17, and 20).

17. C: Participant 7 received a total of 7 points; all the others received 6 points.

18. G: The average age at the time of death for those with 7 close relationships is 14.5 ((13 + 16)/2).

19. B: The oldest baboon was 18 at time of death, and had 9 close relationships. (Baboon 5)

20. G: The youngest baboon at time of death was 3, and had 4 close relationships. (Baboon 4)

21. C: The baboon who lived to be 16 had 7 close relationships. (Baboon 10)

22. J: Baboon 11 has 10 close relationships.

23. D: We know from the premise of the passage that bats can both fly and echolocate.

24. F: The second paragraph states that the long fingers and keeled breastbone suggest that the bat could fly.

25. B: Scientists did not find features around the ears that modern day bats use to echolocate.

26. J: Olfactory means related to the sense of smell.

27. C: The scientists estimated the fossil's age by dating the rock formation in which it was found.

28. H: The fossilized bat has more claws than modern bats, which suggests that the bat was a skilled climber.

29. C: According to the first sentence, caffeine may reduce beta amyloidal.

30. H: The mice received the equivalent of 5 8-ounce cups of coffee, or 5 x 8 = 40 ounces of coffee.

31. A: Paragraph 3 lists the benefits of caffeine as treatment; entering the blood stream easily is not listed.

32. H: According to paragraph 2, half the mice, or 50%, received no caffeine.

33. C: The first sentence notes that beta amyloid is a protein.

34. H: The second paragraph notes that the mice were at an age equivalent to 70 years in a human.

35. C: The first sentence of paragraph 2 notes that the device weighs about 1.6 kilograms. The first sentence of paragraph 3 notes that tests have shown it requires little extra metabolic power to produce energy.

36. G: Paragraph 2 notes that the device gets its energy from the energy put into slowing down the knee.

37. C: The first sentence of paragraph 2 notes that the device can generate an average of five watts of electricity.

38. H: The backpack battery is not mentioned as something the device could help power.

39. D: The last sentence of the passage notes that scientists are working on making the device smaller and more lightweight.

40. F: The last sentence of paragraph 2 notes that the concept is similar to that used by hybrid-electric cars.

Post Exam

After the exam, when you've had the time to rest and relax from the stress you put your brain through, take the time to critically evaluate your test performance. This will help you gain valuable insight into how you performed and what sort of score you should be expecting.

Remember, this is neither an opportunity to over-inflate your ego, nor to put yourself down. The main idea is to make your self-evaluation objective and critical, so that you will achieve an accurate view of how things will pan out.

This doesn't mean that you should begin a session of "if only I'd…" or "I shouldn't have…" This will only depress you. The point of this exercise is to keep you grounded, open minded and optimistic.

Soon enough, you'll receive your score, so remain optimistic and patient and hopefully it will exceed your expectations!

Made in the USA
San Bernardino, CA
22 December 2015